SMALL IMPORTANT THINGS

*Spiritual Fiction for the
Emerging Man*

Paul Broomfield

BALBOA.
PRESS

A DIVISION OF HAY HOUSE

Balboa Press books may be ordered through booksellers or by contacting:

Balboa Press
A Division of Hay House
1663 Liberty Drive
Bloomington, IN 47403
www.balboapress.com
1 (877) 407-4847

Because of the dynamic nature of the Internet, any web addresses or
links contained in this book may have changed since publication and
may no longer be valid. The views expressed in this work are solely those
of the author and do not necessarily reflect the views of the publisher,
and the publisher hereby disclaims any responsibility for them.

The author of this book does not dispense medical advice or prescribe the use
of any technique as a form of treatment for physical, emotional, or medical
problems without the advice of a physician, either directly or indirectly. The
intent of the author is only to offer information of a general nature to help
you in your quest for emotional and spiritual well-being. In the event you use
any of the information in this book for yourself, which is your constitutional
right, the author and the publisher assume no responsibility for your actions.

Any people depicted in stock imagery provided by Thinkstock are
models, and such images are being used for illustrative purposes only.
Certain stock imagery © Thinkstock.

Printed in the United States of America.

ISBN: 978-1-4525-9462-0 (sc)
ISBN: 978-1-4525-9463-7 (e)

Balboa Press rev. date: 04/09/2014

Preface

In Greek terms the genius was a guardian spirit largely the force of one's natural desires.

I started from a deep sleep with the clearest, most certain vision I have ever had in my life. That clarity of vision was accompanied by a stillness and calm that would make it come into reality. I had the beginning and the end of a story, and all I had to do was fill in the middle. In this instance, either through luck or necessity, I think I was completely surrounded by my genius.

Since that epiphany moment over 4 years ago I have become expert in a few things, not least of which is my own futility in bringing things into creation. That, of course, is all part of the learning process. Coming face to face with fears, negating patterns, insecurities, doubts and maybe most debilitating of all, excuses. Those are some fierce demons to battle.

I key a "Man" as a:

1. Physical specimen
2. Intellectually learned (Who is also thirsty for more knowledge)
3. Emotionally self-sustainable
4. Spiritually in service

These four components make up what I consider to be a Gentleman.

The journey into and through the initiation of becoming a Man is perilous, tiring and most often unrecognized. In a modern western world uninitiated itself, this makes the journey even more demanding because it means the individual, in most instances, needs to self-initiate himself. It all comes down to one thing for me. The joy of learning. Finding enthusiasm in the challenge and placing faith and consistency into the process will ensure advancement along the long lonely road to becoming an autonomous, wise and compassionate individual.

For any women reading 'Small Important Things' please be gentle when you see/feel/sense an Emerging Man in your midst. The Feminine tendency and gift is to challenge the Masculine, but please know that any male putting himself through a self-initiation is already being challenged in myriad ways by an archaic paradigm. It is a fragile time. Your support (Only sometimes mind you, it is not to say that the challenges are not needed or unwarranted) will be soothing to a raw part of this man, and give a sense of nourishing acknowledgment that may just do enough to keep him pointing in the direction of becoming a Man who husbands, stewards and protects the Sacred Divine Feminine, which is the Masculine tendency and gift.

If you have a man in your life that would benefit from this story then please share it with them. Females have a more accepted avenue of expressing themselves emotionally within a group of others, and it's my hope that this tale will give tools to a male with few resources at his disposal to continue and to amplify his emotional maturation.

Finally, with my genius, I have brought about 'Small Important Things' to not only educate, but also to open up a discussion on redefining the "Modern Man." A Modern Man archetype that is more closely akin to the Renaissance or Gentle Man. To a Man capable, assured, wise and compassionate, rather than that of the stooge, bully, incompetent, or fool.

That in some future reflection I can look upon my effort with pride and nostalgia knowing that I truly tried my best. I humbly offer it to you that it may bless your path.

It is every male's birthright to come into Manhood.

Dedication

To the Sacred Feminine who has inspired me into becoming a better Man. And to all of my Teachers along my path that are helping me to reach and be worthy of the mantle of Manhood and the Divine Grace of God. Specifically Shree Shivkrupand Swami, Paramahansa Yogananda, Wade McKinley, Joseph Campbell, Yogi Vishvaketu, Dr. Madan Bali, Bobby Campo, Bryce Nagels and Benjamin Ribkoff.

Contents

Chapter 1: **Ding Dong**

Ding Dong.

There was the customary 30-second pause that comes after the doorbell rings. Then the vibrations and shift in air pressure as the occupant comes to unlatch the lock and open the door.

"Yes?"

"I'm the teacher you've been asking for."

This was the first time they had ever met.

...If clarity had a colour... He thought. A slight spontaneous laugh escaped his mouth as he asked the very reasonable question.

"I'm sorry, do I know you?"

"Yes." There was a seemingly permanent natural smile on his face.

A pause of a few seconds began to lengthen. The eyes of the guest held calm and unwavering as the discomfort and awkwardness of the man's grew. The novelty of the situation started to wane for him with that silence. The spontaneity of the laughter turned into a nervous sputtering.

"Uhh...ok...uhm, and how do I know you?"

Another slight pause, perhaps four seconds, but it felt an eon for the man as he fidgeted and made a thousand unconsciously conscious movements.

It was a beautiful condo. Dark stone façade, recently renovated, but keeping intact the early 20th century character. Cast iron railings with intricate foliage patterns leading to the front door, a deep fire engine red. Purchased by the owner because he thought that a home should have a red door as its entryway. Plus, it was the only house on the block to have the distinction. A distinction he took a strange and subtle pleasure from. Overlooking Parc LaFontaine in Montreal's Plateau Mont-Royal, it also had the distinction of being in one of the trendiest areas in town.

The four seconds were stifling to the man. His grip to the inside handle of the door had grown vice-like.

"That clear calling in your mind that resonates guidance and protection, even when everything else around and inside you seems to be drowning in confusion. Just as you know that voice and clear calling with fullness and trust, you know me."

You could have heard a pin drop in his mind. For the briefest, most beautiful of moments, there was silence in his head. There was space. There was soothing respite from the constant deluge that was relentless in his mind. It was, however, only the briefest of moments.

Chapter 2: Daniel History

Daniel was an above average, average guy. Adept at any number of sports, his body just seemed to know the movements required of him. A hand-eye coordination unpracticed, and because of the normalcy of the adaptability it provided, largely unnoticed by him.

Same said for almost every facet and aspect of his formative and adolescent years. Above average, average. Able to get by with this capacity he was seldom called on or challenged to tap a deeper sense of commitment.

In a way, this lack of pressure had allowed for a lovely sense of innocence. A natural and kind way of being in presence with others. With an endearing, and somewhat ignorant subtlety, Daniel would make whomever he was with feel as though he was truly with them. This gift, well above average, was a main component in his successes later on in life. When his large brown eyes had focused intently upon someone, it was neither intense nor poignantly focused. There was simply allowance and a soft listening held within his gaze. One was not alone with those eyes.

And so Daniel was rarely alone. It was a commodity much sought after by those in his circle of influence. It suited him to be the social chameleon, because within the confines of a conversation about someone else, he need not think of himself. Nor of the ache and hole that was perpetually present.

Daniel had moved to Montreal six years earlier from London, Ontario. "It's Montreal" he thought at the time.

The more refined sense of elegance. To experience the North American anomaly of a big city under the influence of a different culture and language.

For Daniel there was coarseness in his hometown. The need to step beyond long held boundaries and the feeling of routine. As though he could see the inevitability of becoming a big fish in a small bowl. Montreal was a safe bet. Far enough away to have his space, close enough to fulfill family obligations when needed, and still in Canada.

A second generation Canadian family, the Shaughnessy's did everything by the book, and expected their offspring to do the same. Christmas and Thanksgiving was turkey dinner, Boxing Day shopping, Canada Day was park picnics, stick on tattoos, and a massive bowl of potato salad.

"It never gets eaten." Was Daniel's annual statement. And it never did. It sat with a massive wooden spoon, to match the proportion of the bowl, protruding at a gravity-defying angle. Getting the gradual coating of toughness, which is the fate of any untouched pudding or mashed dish. All the while, popsicles, pop, and beer cans were fetched from the green Coleman cooler situated below the bowl.

The expectations of his parents to tow the line were not lacking in love. The rules were liberal, but also distinct for "his own good." The expectations were to fit into the mould of the Canadian middle class.

And while Daniel definitely felt loved and accepted by his family, he did not feel understood. This sense that his parents or younger sister did not really know him was another catalyst in the move to the island.

CHAPTER 1(A): Ding Dong Ya Dingdong

"What are you looking at?!" After the brief moment of calm, the reaction was defensive and caustic. As though with the formless space of that quietude, an elastic band was pulled to it's fullest taut capacity and unleashed with that oscillating "Twwangggggg" vibration.

"I'm looking at you."

"Well why?!"

"Because you are whom with which I am speaking." The logic and simplicity of the response soothed and irritated him all in the same instant. As too did the proper usage of the word "whom". His mother used to correct him every time his grammar was inappropriate. He could hear her voice now, drawing out the end of the word "Whom, whooommmmmm". It was something that at the time bothered him to no end, but now served as a basis for his own eloquence when dealing with clients and colleagues. Language and its symbols are powerful tools.

"But who are you?!"

"I've already told you that. Would you like me to repeat it?"

"No… no I don't, but… why are you here?" He knew his questions were redundant, even while he was asking them he felt himself drowning and grasping in his own thoughts. In complete unison with the guest's response was his own voice in his head saying "He told me that also."

"Who put you up to this? Jared, did Jared make you do this?" Peering around the corner of the doorway, he was thinking he might see a laughing face on the sidewalk, or perhaps behind a tree across the street.

"No one put me up to this. Not in the sense that you're speaking of anyway."

"Why are you being so evasive?"

"I am not being evasive, you are simply not asking the necessary questions."

"Well what if I asked you to get the hell out of here?" He did not want to ask this question. Not now.

"I am not into the game of brinksmanship. My diplomacy is one of being honest and truthful within the confines of the moment, and being respectful of that truth for the sake of everyone involved. I know it is not feasible to expect others to live up to this ideal but it does not change the fact that I expect others to live up to their word. So to answer your question, I would leave if you asked me to leave." Pausing... "Might I say, however, that you don't want to ask me that." His smile got much more playful as he said that last part.

The temperamental side of Daniel felt the frustration of a child wrestling with a teenager. Outmatched and red in the face. Pout lips and the downward gaze of not getting their own way.

The piece soothed by this man's presence was in a hammock swaying between two palm trees. The sun beating down filtered by the palm fronds. An ever so slight breeze coming off the water, and the soft side to side rhythm of the cradle giving allowance for there to be no where else.

Daniel was nowhere else. Enamored, overwhelmed, calm and in love with this man. Easily and without fear, although not every part of him knew it.

These Paul Newman eyes. Alight and playfully mischievous. Cartoonish in their animation. Engendering a feeling of safety, a funneling of another world, that colour of clarity was also the colour of understanding and acceptance. It was the colour of someone who knew.

"You're just a kid. How old are you?!" Incredulous, his tantrum child still had fight left in him.

"I'm 31 years old." The fact that they were the same age was something else that created a tug of war within his mind. Chaffing and soothing.

"And you're capable of teaching me?"

"I am."

"You know I'm getting pretty sick of these short succinct answers."

Silence. And once again that smile of tranquility.

"What are you looking at?! Wait! Wait, I know, I know, you're looking at me. But why don't you say more to me?"

"The reason I have said so little is because your mind is moving exponentially more quickly than my own. If I was to start trying to talk to you at the pace with which your thoughts are moving, it would be like a pedestrian trying to have a conversation with the driver of the speeding car that's going past him on the highway. In short, it would be crazy." As he said this, a large grin crossed his face. A small bubbling giggle jumped from his heart, as though he were laughing at the joke at the expense of craziness. "And so I am simply waiting and hoping for you to apply the brakes. I would very much like to say more to you."

Chapter 2(a): Daniel History X

There are two formative incidents from childhood that formed much of Daniel's personality later on in life. Whether or not he knew it consciously (he didn't) these were the moments that cauterized his wild nature and shackled the powerful and very innocent strength to achieve.

They happened within months of each other in the third grade. His above average intelligence landing him in an accelerated program on top of the regular curriculum. His assignment had been to make a 30-word word-search puzzle for the class. On dinosaurs. Man did he like dinosaurs. He worked on it with verve until he got to word 29 and then he just couldn't think of another. Literally could not fathom of one more word. He racked his brain, and then feared what would happen if he didn't hand it in. Because it was an "all or nothing" thing to his little mind. An 8-year olds imagination can think of a lot of fearful outcomes, but somehow handing in a 29-word word-search when it was asked to be 30 was incomprehensible.

The day the assignment was due he walked into his class tentative and expectant of a reprimand. Some embarrassing spectacle in front of the entire classroom. A Little Reggie look-a-like straight out of the Little Archie comics. And what happened? Nothing. Nothing happened. Not that day or any subsequent. Who knows what would have happened if the teacher had have made mention of it, had have laughed and told him to hand in the 29-word project? Or gotten angry or disappointed at his failure? Instead, the imprint was that it didn't really matter. Either way it didn't matter. This one outcome, or lack of one as the case may be, brought our young hero's enthusiasm to a slow grinding halt. Cue coasting through school doing just enough to get by... now.

Chapter 1(b): **I said "Ding DONG!!"**

It is easy to read and watch situations from a slight distance. Set aside from a conversation for instance, it is a simple observation process to view the varying emotions being expressed by the participants. If Daniel could have watched a video of his conversation with the visitor up to this point, he would have been amazed to see just how much he was fidgeting. He would have seen his eyes darting, darting, darting, from spot to space and back again. And he would have seen, in contrast to his own movements, the stable stillness of the man standing on his front step.

It was not that Daniel was fearful or afraid of this man, in fact, from the first he felt an inherent trust. It's just that holding eye contact with this man for any longer than 2 or 3 seconds spooked his insides. As though his interior were being exposed to a light and it had forgotten to put some clothes on. His insides, for lack of a better term, were bashful.

"That space that I had spoken of earlier has always been present for you. The deep and subtle feeling that you are the centre of your life is no lie. The unspoken secret that since childhood you have kept to yourself. You know, the one that you are the epicenter of the entire universe… that's true."

"What are you talking about?"

"I'm speaking of you being chosen. This is life giving you a wake up call."

"My wake up call is a 31 year-old surfer dude claiming to be my teacher?"

"Just think of me as your own personal Mr. Myagi Daniel-san"

CHAPTER: Day to Day Sidetrack

The metro was a haven for Daniel. He felt a sense of anonymity in the train. A feeling of safety. There was little to no attachment with the fellow riders of the orange or green lines. Just a constant rotation of fresh faces, and new people needing to "go" somewhere.

It was not uncommon for Daniel to walk to Sherbrooke station and ride the train for what he had dubbed to himself as a "circuit". Taking the orange line to Snowden, transferring to the blue line to get to Jean Talon, and then connecting back onto the southbound orange to return to Station Mont Royal, and walk back to his place. Generally it would take a little over an hour to make it door to door. In that time it allowed him the freedom to sit back and watch people, read a book, listen to music, but mostly, and perhaps most importantly for him, to write. Getting out of the house and moving was a catalyst for his inspiration.

Sherbrooke was like a launching pad out of the Battlestar Gallactica T.V. series. Standing on the south end platform overlooking the tracks, were giant white (aged and yellowed a touch) tiled walls, and the darkness of the tunnel leading out into the depths of space. It was sometimes a little shattering to the fantasy when the round bulbous blue worm of the train came through the tube.

Coming full circle into the earthy and hearth-like station of Mont Royal, it was his favourite station. Rust coloured and brown bricks, there was something that suited his previous ideals as to what Montreal would be to him.

Combining the simple warmth of the brick lined walls, the white signage spaced every ten metres stating "Mont-Royal", and the community that the station provided for. It was a fashionable and young area, the plateau. All of it was "his" Montreal.

To Daniel, the Montreal woman dressed extremely well. Achieving a fashion sense that was well put together, but not over done. Flamboyant, yet not garish. Displaying layers and accessories without looking as though she had tried too hard. Put on top of that the Gallic tendency to have full lips and smouldering eyes, and he was hooked. Daniel loved tenacious delicacies.

Before moving to the city, he had heard from a number of friends and sources that Montreal was a city obsessed with sex, and the women were, to put it bluntly (as most friends and sources were apt to do), easy.

It was a claim that he actually found to be quite accurate.

Young, classically tall, dark and handsome, and the confidence of someone well set up in a career with high prospects, the spectacle of Daniel at the bar, be it in one of his suits or simply a pair of jeans and a t-shirt, was sure to attract the attention of one, or several women. And on the odd occasion, for that matter, an interested male party.

CHAPTER PRE-1: Before the Ding Dong

It was a morning begun like any other. Waking up in his bed, Daniel didn't know it, but it was the 11,472nd consecutive day where he was not fearful for his life getting under the covers. 31 years, 5 months, and 7 leap year days, had conditioned him into feeling safe and warm in his delving into dreamtime.

Not to say that he hadn't had his fair share of pre-sleep anxiety, worry, drunken nausea, anxiety driven hyper thoughts, indigestion, horniness, neurotic reconstruction of the previous days events, neurotic construction of the next days events, or even just an inability to close his eyes and drift away. But he had never felt a physical fear for his person. And never having been truly scared for his life, he would wrap himself up in the cinnamon bun of warmth and comfort, and drift away.

Generally upon waking, give or take 2 seconds, Daniel would have 2 seconds of clarity and space before his mind would kick into gear and start the planning of the days events or other such issues. A beautiful space where there were still the vestiges of safety and non-attachment to responsibility.

It was a beautiful queen size. Iron cast frame, (not unlike the railings leading up to the front door), posturepedic mattress, sheets 300 count, down duvet, ergonomic chiropractic pillows. A haven to spend one third of a life.

There was only a brief 1-second respite upon waking this morning. Before the ideas of work and engagements came to rest upon him like a sheet draped over a potted plant. The need and desperate urge to feel productive, while giving a sense of purpose, was stifling to a part of him feeling the need for "more". Of that part feeling the need for "freedom".

That last word can be a grand cliché, over used and over exploited by those trying to over use and over exploit. But for those of us who do not have the sensation of actually being free, to do, and to be, and to choose, there is no cliché. There is just a heart wrenching desire for the release of restrictive yokes.

This was a morning that with the clear chime of some truth resonating (not more loudly, just more broadly), the mind increased it's pitch and battle of it's own war cries. A tactic designed to create distraction and tumult. And from the initial surge came what had been a common lament in the previous year. "Oh God, Why can't this all just cease?"

It was the need for a deeper quietude. Beyond the level of money in the bank, and fitting the mould of a "good catch". In the existential visualization of a mountain lake, mirror-like, reflecting back to the sky and horizon it's own beauty, Daniel did not have first hand experience of this ethereal place. It was still only a concept. A place he had only heard of, or seen on a poster. A mental construct that he needed to be true.

It was answers he was looking for. Daniel was looking for answers.

Chapter 1(c): Yeah That's Right I'm saying Ding Dong Again

"Have you been following me?"

"No I have not."

"Well how do you know my name?"

Clean-shaven and a square jaw, his smile had, seemingly, gotten more wry in the past moment. A smile, Daniel thought, that knew a secret and wanted to spill the beans.

"You need to start understanding that life has symbols. It gives guidance if we slow down and trust it's rhythm. The randomness of life is not so random if you know what you are looking for. My coming here is no mistake. You are ready for a teacher, and I am ready to be of service. This is the sign that you have been waiting for."

"How do you know? I'm actually quite happy." A stranger basically telling you that you're not living your life properly will most definitely bring up indignant responses.

"And I'm certain that a piece of you truly believes that. Just as I am certain that a major part of you right now is violently screaming that I am a crazy kook trying to con you. Or steal from you. Or destroy you. But I am not talking to that part of you, because it is trying to control things through fear. That piece of you that gets defensive and offended at what I say is not viable in this relationship.

I am speaking to your clarity Daniel. From my place of honesty to yours.

I can see that you are aching. Hemorrhaging energy. And that can be so tiring, believe me I know. But this is the time to change that and heal the wounds. It is inefficient to live how you are right now."

"How do you mean "inefficient"?" It was Daniel's habit to always use his fingers as quotation marks. Something he had started when he was in early adolescence because he thought it made him look a bit more intelligent, and hence, older. Now it was something that made him seem geeky or condescending to those he used it with.

"May I come in?"

"Excuse me?" There were red flags popping up all over the place in his head.

"I asked if you would allow me to come into your home."

Daniel's mind raced, ...*I knew it I knew it!! He's a fucking vampire!! He's going to slice your throat! As soon as you invite him across the threshold he can do anything he wants! Don't trust him, you CAN'T trust him!!*...

Everything had exclamation points in his head. Everything was a major dramatic episode at this point. The boundaries of manners and normal proper conduct were the only things preventing him from pushing the man down the stairs, slamming the door shut, and running to call emergency.

And so with a doe-eyed look, scarcely the acme of someone calm and collected, Daniel stepped aside and gave a sweeping motion with his arm. ... *Yeah! Test him! Don't say a word or answer the question!!! That's it!!*...

"You haven't answered my question."

"What?! Oh, right, uhm please come in." …*Shitshitshitshit, he's a vampire! A fucking vampire!!...*

Striding into the hallway and shuffling off his sandals they made eye contact once again.

"Where is your kitchen?"

They walked to the end of the hall and to the left of the dining area where the modern accoutrements of his fully furnished kitchen were.

"Ok, I'll need two glass bowls and a bottle of soya sauce."

Chapter 2(b): Daniel History XX...X

The second incident in his early formative years affected him in much the same way as the first, only instead of dampening a zeal for performance it would be a tourniquet to his love impulse. Not stemming the flow completely, but reducing and mutating its ability to mature. Because this incident came at a time of innocence before hormones had a chance to REALLY fuck things up.

Sat on the yellow bus after school, he had been thinking about it for a couple days. Unable to hold the secret to himself any longer he turned to his friend Mark and confided.

"I think I have the hots for Kirsten." It was a young boys first confidence to a friend that he felt 'different' about someone. A curious, giddy, and new sensation.

Immediately, the girl sat in front of their bench seat turned around. Francine, the tallest girl of their class, the girl who had the odd talent of rolling her tongue back in her mouth and shooting a stream of saliva from the bottom of her mouth, said with a form of zeal bordering on smug antagonism.

"I'm going to tell her." As though that was all she needed to say or do, she turned back to face the front.

It was shocking to him. He didn't know what to do. His face blanched and then blushed. Exposing a boy's first real foray into expressing affection for a girl was hard, brutal even. But sadly this was not where the real damage occurred because what came next rippled through to his future relationships with love and fear. Planting a virulent program into an extremely impressionable mind.

It's the curse of the vast majority of young men in Western Culture, learning love through peers (or God help us, advertising) with incomplete initiations rather than a trusted and experienced mentor/elder.

The implied tattling was bad, but it was nothing in terms of what his friend would say to him next. After a few minutes of silence, with voice a barely audible whisper in order to protect himself, he once again turned to Mark, this time for advice as to what to do. These three words would place his heart in a glass case. Forever on display, never to be touched.

"Just deny it."

Chapter: **Nighttime Rendezvous**

The smoothest of silk skin. Like touching shea butter cream itself.

Liquid chocolate groans. The type that resonates not only from the mouth and throat, but from the bottom of the belly as well.

Combine those forces of nature with the undulating rhythm of hips, torso, and limbs and Daniel was in his playground.

"I am Winnie the Pooh." He thinks.

It is the unselfish service of creating pleasure that is the hallmark of an accomplished lover. The excitement of being part of another's excitement. There are givers and takers in this world, and Daniel wanted to take pleasure from giving.

Within this was also the humility borne of being a bit of a nerd in school. As everyone knows, the geek seldom receives the ardor of affection from the opposite sex. Having the lean times in his formative (and some might say hellish) years of puberty, Daniel learned the blessing of being allowed into the private and sacred realm of a naked woman.

To be in such close palpable vicinity of such a protected and vulnerable place for his partner, was a profound trust not lost on him. And he absolutely loved to feel her opening up despite normal convention.

"You taste amazing." His hands were on her abdomen. All that left her mouth was a barely audible gasp. Her head tilted up and back to the right, eyes closed, feeling and seeing from the inside out. One hand in his hair, and the other close to her own slightly opened pouting mouth. The visual had him stand at attention more and more. It would not be long until they consummated their relationship. It would not be long until the pulse and pump of the dance would take on a new form.

CHAPTER: **Pre-Nighttime Rendezvous**

The pulse and pump of the bar was in full effect. Bar lights and booze make everyone's attractiveness go up a notch. Just how much is subjective to number of cocktails and the seekers level of loneliness.

The mating dance in the nightclub environment is as much a game as what "go fish" is to little children. You've got to demand the right numbers in order to make the pair. People running around asking if anyone's gotten any 4's, 7's, or kings, in the guise of small talk and feigned interest. Match enough cards and chances are someone is not sleeping in their own bed that night.

Daniel had become a bit of a connoisseur of the bar scene. People watching, was after all, a big part of his job. Groups of 3 or more girls he had noticed for example had two types. Type-1, when making their way through the throng, always have the best looking of the group go first. As they snake their way through the dance floor, up to the bar, or towards the bathroom, the farther away from the lead girl you went, generally the more pudgy, portly, or ugly the girls will get. *Bless their hearts* Daniel thought, *they still have the same staunch and snobbery as if they were spearheading the whole group.* Type-2 has the most beautiful go second, with a protective chaperone leading as deterrent to the marauding suitors.

Daniel would always set his sites on the matriarch of the group. He knew what he liked.

"Hi" Every woman has something unique to amplify her beauty. For Jessika, it was her collarbones. The spaghetti strap pink tank top was the perfect compliment to the sleek curvature leading to her soft feminine neck.

"Hi"

"I'm Daniel."

"I'm Jessika."

"Jessika? Is that with a 'C' or a…"

"Oh my god!? No it's with a 'K'! How did you know that!? That is so crazy! No one has ever asked that before. How did you know that?" Something else that her clavicles led to was a thin gold chain and a stylized "Jessika", dangling, just below that lovely indent at the base of her neck.

"You don't look like you'd be a run of the mill Jessica. There's something a little more unique and exotic about you." She laughed and touched his arm. "May I buy you a drink Jessika?"

"Sure I'd love one."

These were the first instances that precipitated the two lying in Daniel's bed that night. That led to Daniel's hands pulling down her sheer panties. That led to the beautiful discovery of a new body. New scents. New sounds.

CHAPTER 1(D): Oh… You Said DING Dong. Right… I Get it Now.

"It's not all going to happen at once you know." He had been making the up and down dolloping action for the past minute. Filling one of the bowls half full of soya sauce.

"What?" Daniel was oddly transfixed by what was transpiring.

"The correct response, Daniel, is 'excuse me' or 'pardon me', and I'm speaking about the trust you feel for me. It's not all going to happen at once."

He had finished with the soya sauce and had filled the remainder of the bowl with water. In the other bowl, he simply filled it with water and placed it beside the one with the dark black mixture.

"The body is designed to succeed. We are supposed to feel good all the time." He dragged out and accentuated the pronunciation of 'all'. "And if we don't feel wonderful all the time, then something is wrong, and it's our responsibility to fix it.

Now the fully-grown body is a wonderful piece of technology. 50 to 100 trillion cells all working in unison to ensure that the organism as a whole continues to function. This intelligence in creation is what makes our eyelashes grow as eyelashes, stomach lining as stomach lining, biceps as biceps. You get the point." Daniel's mouth was slightly agape. "It also provides for the functioning of these cells in the form of blood pressure, digestion, hair growth, hormones et cetera, and the vitalistic healing principles of the body. Which is what these two bowls are here to signify. To understand the vitalistic principles of the body is in many ways to understand how to live a healthy life. An efficient life.

Under the right conditions and proper guidance, the body and it's inhabitant can become an immensely powerful conduit of life.

Under adverse conditions, the body will do anything it can to ensure survival and the perpetuation of its life. Given the choice, the body will always want for the right conditions, and will heal and amplify itself through those times.

Here we have two bowls. This bowl signifies a healthy and vibrant body. It is clear and pure. We can see through it and get information with clarity and ease. This other bowl is a body cluttered and confused with an unhealthy lifestyle. What little light we can make out is dampened and muddied. The information can still get through, but the message is convoluted.

Are you with me?"

Looking from the bowls to his eyes, Daniel was thinking about how much he'd like a glass of water. His mouth was dry and his breathing was quite shallow. An odd familiarity came to him as though he was in a Grade-8 lab experiment.

"Yes, yes I'm with you."

"Good. We take now a drop of soya sauce, what for this analogy is an unhealthy act. For example smoking a cigarette or eating fried fatty food. Watch carefully as I put a drop into the bowl." Holding the bottle a foot above the darkened bowl, a drop dripped into the mixture. "And what did you notice happening to the water?"

"Uh… nothing really."

"That's right, the accumulation of so many other unhealthy acts covers up the effect. Now we add a drop to the clean and clear water, and what happens?"

"It contaminates it."

"The effect of the drop is completely visible. The water is no longer as clear as it was, and the body, that before was able to put it's focus upon other more subtle information, now has to go back to work fixing and making reparations to itself at a physical level.

And it WILL heal itself. This is the natural intrinsic vitalistic quality of the body. It's possible to filter and clean oneself if we cease putting the poisonous drops into the mix. Not convoluting the situation is as simple as making the right choices. It is the efficiency of right living." He stopped, smiled, and placed his hands wide upon the table top. Allowing his straight arms to press his shoulders up towards his ears. Once again silence descended upon the pair.

"I don't smoke." It was all he could think to say. Almost blurting it out in an affirmation of being on the right path. Seeking approval.

"Excellent." He was laughing again. "That's really excellent."

CHAPTER: Day to Day

…Oh no. No no, he's not going to do it, aww no don't, no don't arrrrgggghhhhh, he did it, he totally did it!…

Riding the green line, the train was between the McGill and St. Laurent stations. It was Daniel's reaction every time he witnessed it. Sat on the train it was always on his way home from work that he would see someone doing it.

In the morning people still had their senses about them. They had the strength of a good nights sleep and the morning to prepare for the day. But in the afternoon, people had slogged through the workday, they were worn down by the events of the day, and their defenses of normal etiquette were lacking.

The scenario always inspired within him a weird sense of exhilaration, indignation and exasperation. A strange voyeuristic pleasure in seeing someone thinking that they were getting away with something.

He would see, out of the corner of his eye generally, someone's hand go up to their nose. Normally a thumb to the outside of one of the nostrils or the index finger into the under lip of the nose. This is where the fun for him began. Because he could tell almost immediately if they had caught something by what their facial expression did. The facial expression of "Did anybody see me just do that?" The forehead would rise slightly and their eyes would get a far off glaze to them. They would look out the window, or up to the car's ceiling, or get a sudden interest in one of the posters advertising an art exhibition or college program.

Daniel loved this part. Because as much as they were feigning interest in these innocuous things, they were also scoping around to see if anyone was looking at them. And all the while the person would be rolling the little nugget between their thumb and forefinger. No matter where the eyes went, Daniel could tell that the only thought was about how long to wait until they made their move. It was a funny cat and mouse game that was not at all hard to avoid because they were too wrapped up in what they were doing.

It was never less than 30 seconds. Normally about 45, and on the odd occasion, for those being extra careful, 1 or 2 minutes. But the result was the same.

...Oh no, no no, don't do it, no she's not going to do it, awww no, no don't no don't, arrrrggghhh she totally did it!...

It would be something like a quick look out the window, and while leaning against the ledge, looking as innocently as possible of course, the offending hand would make its way casually, oh so horribly casual, towards the mouth. A discreet brushing of the lips. Or a convenient scratch on the cheek or upper lip gets seen to while the digit does an adept fly by to make the deposit.

From there, the lips purse, and the face, relieved by the completion of the mission, also hides a slight shame in having picked their nose and eaten it in public.

Daniel shared this shame. He felt the flush of embarrassment in having taken part in the production. But for him it was like seeing an accident, he just couldn't stop himself from watching.

He could also do nothing but be a bystander. Even thinking of saying something, or intervening with a tissue, immobilized his insides and tightened his stomach muscles with fear.

So he sat or stood, face sedate and unflinching, showing none of the emotion bubbling below the surface.

CHAPTER: **Nighttime Rendezvous by Daylight**

The sun was shining through the window. Early morning light, clear and sharp, with the backdrop of the sky a translucent blue.

Her eyes were still shut, mouth slightly open to allow the long full breaths of sleep an easy passage.

Daniel had been up for the past half an hour just watching her. In this peace and quiet she looked like a little child, snuggled up safe and sound under the covers. Every once in a while her nose would scrunch up or a small spastic twitch would course through her face. In many ways it was a perfect moment. Tranquil, sweet and serene.

In the time of watching the bare little cherubim, there was only one thought going through his head. "When is she going to get out of here?" Hair that was golden last night was mousy this morning. Skin that glowed now had spots and hairs growing in conspicuous places. And an energy he had tried so vigorously to get together with was now, in every aspect, a repulsion.

It had nothing to do with Jessika. Just as it had nothing to do with Sophie, or Amelie, or Sarah, or Jennifer, or Jennifer, or Marie Claude.

It was the proximity with which they had come to. He couldn't get away from the feeling that he was going to lose something. A claustrophobic sensation of having his freedom threatened.

She yawned, stretched and smacked her lips a couple times. Slowly her eyes opened as she hugged the pillow.

"Good morning." She said. A soft whispering perkiness to contrast the sheer bounciness of the night previous. Her eyes met his.

"Hi." There is only so much discomfort one can hide, no matter how well practiced.

"I had an amazing sleep last night."

"That's good."

"How did you sleep?"

"Good."

"Is everything alright?"

"Yeah."

"Okaaaay, uhm, do you wanna get some breakfast? I know a great little place on St. Denis and Rachel."

"No thanks, I've got a really busy day today."

And that, if you didn't notice it, was where the fracture occurred. The point at which whatever positives, whatever advancements, or connections, or good will they had made, were shattered. Because while the celebration of love can be made in an instant, the same can be said of the dissolution of that trust.

Daniel's heart was already well entrenched behind fortifications and neuroses to notice the shift and shrinking of his past love. And she was past. Even though she was lying beside him looking at his face, there was an estrangement that neither one of them would talk about.

Chapter 1(e): The Ding Dong Challenge

They made eye contact again. The skittishness at the front door had diminished significantly, and Daniel was able to watch for a bit longer the eyes of this blue-eyed Sesame Street character. Smiling behind a kitchen countertop up to his abdomen, it was as though, any second, he would welcome Grover or Elmo onto the set and into the conversation about soya sauce and good living.

"What all these little drops add up to is a gradual disconnection to the present moment, until the poisons and bad habits themselves become a part of the process. A band of loud, brash and abrasive hungry ghosts all calling for what they want. A chorus of selfishness disinterested in the greater good. So while everyone has the strength and clarity to be strong and clear, these accumulated detriments also have a vote, and until someone realizes their destructive powers, they will be, in one way or another, at the whim of their vote and persuasions."

"In what way?"

"Let me answer that question with a question. What is better for you, an apple and a glass of water, or a bag of cheesy Doritos and a can of Coke?" Daniel laughed a bit at this and wondered if it was a rhetorical question.

"The apple and the glass of water."

"Of course it is, but that doesn't stop people from choosing improperly. Until they are almost impelled by their urges and impulses to disregard their health. And the amazing thing is that these poisons will begin to convince the weakened inhabitant of the body that they will be happier if they take more of what is actually depleting their life." He started to pour the contents of the bowls into the sink. "I've noticed that you didn't say anything about fried fatty foods."

"Excuse me?"

"That's better. You told me that you don't smoke, but you didn't say anything about fried fatty foods."

Daniel didn't know why, but he felt like a child who just had the brilliant plan of stuffing everything under the bed, and saying that the room was clean, exposed.

"Well that's because I still do have some." He said it with a pinch of arrogance and impetuous pride. "… You know… once in a while." And that with a tinge of regretting apology.

"That's alright. There's no judgment about what you've done in the past. It's over, and now we go forward. But from now on you won't be having any more."

"Hmph, excuse me?" The spasm of Daniel's face was immediate, like he had just smelled a bad fart.

"DANIEL!!" His voice clapped liked thunder, and Daniel gave a noticeable start. For the first time the stranger's eyes blazed beyond peace and compassion. "If you wish to challenge me, please come up with something more original and mature than ignorant indignation! You clearly heard what I said. That is the fourth time you have feigned not heard me, as though using it as some stalling tactic. It is nothing but a waste of both of our time. I had stated that you will no longer be eating fried fatty foods. Until you have the strength and wisdom to make proper decisions for yourself, I will make them for you."

"Well, that's just it, who made you king over me?"

"I am not a king over you. It is actually the exact opposite. You are the king in training. I am your teacher. And to answer your question, life made that decision for us."

"You keep on talking about life as though it is some sentient entity with knowledge as to what it's doing and why it's doing it."

"And what do you think it is?"

He had never thought of it in those terms. It was a question that handcuffed his mind and creased his forehead.

Daniel looked out the window to the shining summer day. It was green and lush wherever there were not buildings or the blue sky.

For a moment his gaze rested on a brown throated thrush perched on the fence. With the windows closed he could just make out the muffled song as the feathered chest made almost imperceptible movements.

Daniel got up and opened a couple of the windows. It was the first natural thing he had done in the last twenty minutes. The first wave of fresh air splashed him in the face. He sobered up with that breeze. He turned to the man that he didn't know, but who he had felt an odd kinship with.

"So what now? You say you're here to "teach" me," (Again with the finger quotations) "but what does that mean? How much money are we talking about here?" … *he probably wants a fortune…* "How much time is this going to take?" … *I've got a lot of important things to do I can't lose my freedom to do all the things I have to do because I already have so many other things that need to be done…* "And what about…"

"Daniel just stop. Stop. Slow down for a second. Take a deep inhale… and now a releasing exhale. You've asked some valid questions there, so let's answer those.

First of all, this all works within proximity and constancy. The lessons will not have the same effect if separation of time and space go beyond a certain limit.

In terms of money, I do not want, nor do I need any money from you. It is not the reason that this is being done.

And finally, in terms of time? I can not be certain of that because it is all dependant upon your level of openness and commitment."

"An indeterminate amount of time with proximity and constancy? What does that mean?"

"It means that I move into your home and we begin your tutelage immediately."

Bang! Crash! Biff! Jork! The long held aristocracy in Daniel's mind did not like this one bit. And they had been taking the Batman-esque power punches since this STRANGER (They wanted that description capitalized and in bold) arrived on the scene. Sure they were fat and lazy and arrogantly privileged, but they were also quite happy to be all of those things. They were not so willing to give up control.

"Whoa. Whoa. Whoa. I don't know if that's a good idea. I don't even know who you are. I don't know where you come from. I don't even know your name for god's sake."

"Ok Daniel, we'll have a little challenge. If I win, I will move in with you and you can know what my name is, and as we progress, you can know all of the relevant details of my life that will be of aid to yours." He stopped, smiled, and took a huge releasing breath.

Chapter 3: It Begins

Anyone looking at Daniel on the metro this morning could easily see that he was embroiled in a mental battle of black cloud proportions. Generally speaking, most people on public transit have the cautionary disaffected look of no emotion. Which, of course, belies the fact that they are trying to hold the ocean back with a push broom. But even in that state, people are still aware of those surrounding them, acutely sensitive to minor shifts or body movement.

Daniel, though, was entrenched. Oblivious to those around him, it made the spectacle of him even more conspicuous. Three piece suit with sharp shoes looking so disheveled and distant. The creases on his forehead and the furrow on his brow, with a 5 o'clock shadow at 9 in the morning, gave him a strange dynamic.

It is an unnerving sensation to be completely ignored by someone, even if it is for a brief instant. Some of the people to have taken note of Daniel had thoughts like "Geez… rough weekend." And "I'm glad I don't feel like that guy."

Autopilot. His moves were mechanical. Walking routine train tracks down the street he had walked for the previous six years. Into the building and up the elevator, (His normal guilty voice that said he should walk up the stairs to the office was silent today) across the threshold of the office, and straight into his own private space. Door closed, he had been sitting in his chair for the past three hours looking out his 4th floor window at the downtown scene.

Replaying arguments and hypothetical scenarios over and over since the previous days events. A continuous, tedious, monotonous game of tennis that had been going on since the door closed and the challenge had begun.

The challenge set out before him was a simple one. The stranger would be placed in the spare room of the condo. A seal would be taped across the doorframe and whoever broke the seal would be the loser.

"What do I get if I win?" there was a peaked interest being restrained in his voice as he asked this.

"Nothing. You get nothing Daniel. If I lose the challenge I will walk out of your house and out of your life. You will receive nothing." The voice, posture, and space around him when he said this was without emotion. No smile. No reassuring glow. Daniel glimpsed, for a brief instant, a void and distance that frightened him.

They went up to the room, the stranger making a stop in the bathroom beforehand. Then he simply walked into the room, sat down on the ground, and crossed his legs. The procession leading up to the room and the man sitting down, seemed to Daniel, to be silent and somber. Almost like an execution. As soon as he sat down, however, the glow had returned to the visitors face, and the last words out of his mouth to Daniel had been ringing in his head ever since.

"One should uphold oneself by the Self; one should not degrade oneself; for the Self alone can be a friend to oneself, and the Self alone can be an enemy of oneself." He paused, smiled, and then told Daniel to close the door with a firmness and finality that punched him in the heart.

The old man had been walking from garbage can to garbage can for the past five minutes. Clad in the typical outfit of someone who does not regularly take a shower. Every article having an earthiness to it. Even if he was wearing a piece of clothing with colour on it, other than brown or army green, it would have homogenized itself into the bland colour spectrum of dirt, sweat and smoke. A brown throated thrush.

From garbage can to garbage can, an awkward shuffling gait, shoulders hunched, and back bowed. Head tilted slightly to the left. And while his right hand searched the garbage cans, in his left hand was a freshly bought deli sandwich. The bread and fresh vegetables were out of place in contrast to the man. Like seeing a bright happy balloon floating around in post-apocalyptic earth.

All attention seemed to be placed into the garbage and what treasures might lay hidden within. But the left hand would move continually, mechanically, towards the mouth. Bite after unchewed bite being stuffed into his face. The sandwich could have been anything, a cupcake, a piece of pizza, play-doh. It was only filling space. It was grotesque. A sad and ugly scene.

Daniel's face reflected the pity and fear of witnessing the old vagrant. Pity for the fact that he doubted whether the old man would ever find what he was looking for. Or even, for that matter, whether he would know it if he did actually find it.

The fear was stemming from the fact that within the feeling of pity, there was the growing sense of reflection, that he was not far removed from this man. That he was in a fruitless search. Like this man, he was in a fruitless search. That he was in a fruitless search.

...I am one step away from being that man...

The bottom dropping out was instantaneous. Sprinting out of the office like a diarrhea sufferer runs for the bathroom. The colleagues who had before been whispering about his strange conduct, now had more fodder for the fire.

It was a frantic charge down the stairs. It was a frantic everything. Bursting out of the recycled air of the building, he nearly knocked over the old man he had been watching just seconds earlier. In the brushing by of his catalyst he received a whiff of stale alcoholic breath and urine, with a stink-face look that would have had one believe that Daniel was the crazy one, and the old man was the archetype of one in complete control of his situation and faculties.

... There's no way he's still there. It's been a whole day. There's no way. I'm sorry, I'm so sorry. Please be there, please...

If Daniel was a sight on his way to work this morning, then he was an outright flashing marquee in his rush to get back home.

In total it was close to 22 hours since he had taped the signed sheet of paper across the doorframe, and begun his insane battle of what to do. 22 hours. 22 hours of thinking about not thinking about this man and the scenario.

Pride is an extremely strenuous and demanding exercise. It seeps in to taint and colour all thoughts. Making even the most commonplace actions coarse and unbearable.

Daniel, since closing the door, had done everything intentionally loud and unintentionally clumsy. Music was pumping, television on, even for the first time in weeks he vacuumed. Whatever was started was eventually abandoned when it did not have the desired effect. A tragic clown doing nothing but fooling himself. The realization that had been in the making was simple and shocking.

Daniel was alone. Everywhere he went, no matter how many people might have been around him, there was a bitter black hole.

He was out of breath by the time he got to the front door. As hard as it had been for Daniel to awaken to his desolation, it was hand in hand with the, albeit slow, downturn of his health.

The wheezing blood flavoured breaths in his chest, the heightened sympathetic overload of his nervous system, the shaking and fragile grasp of the keys in the lock, all of these things might have been uncomfortable, but there was also exhilaration in his eyes. Part of him was enjoying this like a child in his first roller coaster ride.

His front door was more red. He felt the change of air pressure upon entering his house. And while his physical and mental body were moving faster than what they had been in all of the previous days events, there was something in his emotional form that was unlabored.

There was still uncertainty at the top of the stairs as to whether he was still there or not. The scared voice saying "Please" over and over again.

Abandoning or avoiding ones love is an action that no one ever becomes immune to. Be it something small like not smiling at a stranger, or a grand deception like the one Daniel had been perpetrating up until this point. All of those avoidances add up into debt and burden.

Daniel had no idea what he would do if the man was not there. He could see only darkness and destruction if that was the case. There was nothing beyond that but his own loneliness.

The cursory glance showed that the door had remained untouched. Bursting through the door assuaged all of his paranoid fears and for the first time in the last day he took a deep surging breath. Daniel then broke into huge heaving weeping. Wave after wave of nausea and remorse in an ebb and flow of pent up emotion. Bubbles and billows of snot and mucous. Heart wrenching primal sounds that only death could make. This percolating agony, this beautiful and pitiful sight, was the graceful state of collapse.

He had let Daniel convulse and spew his pain for at least twenty minutes. Never touching him, but always present. When the final fragments had wended their way out in the form of sobs, he placed his hand upon his shoulder.

Daniel raised his head like a knight after the placement of the sword. Awake, present, and clear, he looked up as one with purpose. The inner fire was once more his own.

There was not much said. Most of the communication was slow and caressing to a still tender environment.

At two in the afternoon, after one of the most grueling 24 hour periods of his life, Daniel went into his bedroom, got under the covers in the clothing he had worn all day, top button undone, tie loosened, and immediately fell into an all encompassing slumber.

Bums and babies. That's who else had a sleep like Daniel that night. Face smushed and neck placed at an ungodly angle, but with such a distant and pudgy serenity. Untroubled by lights, movement, or noises. Whether it be true or not that a virtuous man sleeps deep, Daniel lay unconcerned by vice or virtue.

Chapter 3(a): The Other Side

What for Daniel had been a form of hell, for our placid friend had been one of the nicest days possible. There was nowhere to be except where he was. Nothing to do, save for that of sitting and being.

It was a wager made intentionally to play into his strengths. The Siddhartha-like nature of sitting, waiting, and fasting. There were no expectations for the simple fact that he had already accepted that the best he could do was his best. Whether Daniel came around within that time was not up to him. And so, with a warm exuding zeal he sat and waited.

The same time had elapsed for the two, but the description of the frequency and vibration of silence is gross in its deficiencies. Infinite, immortal, immutable and eternal, silence and stillness is a vast land to explore. And it is exactly in that vein, why this man was so content.

Chapter 4: **Routine**

"Rise and shine early bird." His face was no farther than a foot away when Daniel opened his eyes. The pasty dryness in his mouth and throat would only allow for an audible sound close to that of a toilet gurgling. "Just because you've had a release of life doesn't mean that life has stopped to admire your accomplishment. There's work to be done." Towel in hand, there was a ridiculously awake energy around him for six in the morning. "From what I understand of your routine, you need to be out of the house by 9:15. We'll take it a bit softer this morning because it's all so fresh to you, but this is the best time to shed the skins of sleep and make preparations for the day. I'm lighting a fire under your ass here, let's advance on the day!" saying this he threw the towel to cover Daniel's face. "Triple S Daniel, get at 'er."

"Triple S?"

"Shit, shower, shave."

"Oh." A light smile and a corresponding groggy laugh had him roll out of bed and walk into the bathroom. Looking in the mirror, he leaned on the sink to marvel at his reflection... *My God, I look a thousand years old...* suit wrinkled like a crumpled piece of carbon paper, 5 o'clock shadow now a three day growth, and complexion the lighter side of ash.

He took a long breath and began to undress. Purposefully slow, peeling off layers more subtle than shirts and underwear

Looking back to his naked frame in the mirror, he felt the ugly flush of shame at what he had let happen to it. There was just simply a little "more" everywhere. Even though there was no one to watch him, his head had been downcast almost continuously since he removed his clothing.

… How did I let it get to this?…

He knew the answer. Having lived the slippery slope with friends and coworkers, Daniel was still one of the "healthy" ones of his circle. This level of health was of dubious standards.

Hand on the tiled wall of the shower, he stood, head bowed, and let the water run over his face. Mouth slightly open, eyes slightly closed, the warmth and fluid movement kept him immobile. Feeling the cascades come together at his low lip and chin to waterfall into the drain.

… What the fuck have I been doing with my life?…

There was the feeling of incredulous alertness and an odd weight of fatigue at the polar ends of his spectrum.

A banging on the bathroom door brought him out of his reverie. His mind had still been racing, but because of the different angle his thoughts had been coming from, it was like he was exploring a garden with new scents and landscaping.

"Let's go buddy, we have work to do."

"Yeah, ok." the cobwebs were coming loose and dangling "I'm on it." The remainder of his wash became a quick soap and rinse.

Daniel had once had a lady tell him that watching a man shave was one of the most beautiful things she could witness. Saying that the intensity of attention he would place upon himself was unlike anything else. Her statement had imprinted upon him. One of those passing casual statements that arise whenever the act is made, but for some reason bookmark themselves in your psyche.

And it could have been due to the fact that when she said it, her eyes had been gazing just over his right shoulder in the mirror. Naked breasts stroking the still wet skin of his middle torso. Delicate hands moving from the arch of his low back, around the sides of his abdomen, and then slowly, achingly slow, under the towel about his waist. Giving his muscles those beautiful sensitive convulsions of sexual expectation and spasms of tender tickling. It could have been a lot of things to make him enjoy shaving a little bit more. The imprint of nostalgia.

CHAPTER 4(A): **Routine Meditation**

"Some of the changes we make will be immediate, and, if you allow it, relatively painless." He was standing at the kitchen counter with a pile of bags and boxes in front of him. "This stuff, for example, which you used to consider food will now no longer be given the distinction of that honour." The sweeping motion of his arm was intentionally theatrical. "But we're getting ahead of ourselves here. We're normally going to meditate inside in the morning, but today we're going to sit on your front step… old man style!" he had a really big grin when he said this.

"Old man style?"

"That's right, old man style"

"What is that exactly?"

"Daniel you've been so embroiled in the ridiculous nature of your microcosmic life, that you've forgotten the true marvel of the cosmos. Your life is a symphony of awareness. So we're going to sit and listen to what Pythagoras referred to as 'The Celestial Spheres'. Have a seat Daniel my boy, for the next fifteen minutes we're going to be old men in training. Just sitting and watching the world go by. I'm going to give you just one tip, listening is a reception. There is no force or work needed in order to let the world speak to you."

On the top step, in front of the red door they sat. Michaelangelo clouds of white and grey, yellow and peach, fronted the early morning sky. Birds and squirrels had already begun their workday. Songs and chirping in a lighter way. Lush greens, shade upon shade moving as though dancing. Silence amidst the sounds of nature, while all around him at any one time it all seemed to be... breathing. What is there to write about awe?

Chapter 4(b): **Routine Cuppa**

"twwwwweeeeEEEEEEEEEE..."

"Kettle's boiling." Daniel would come to learn that he said this every time the kettle would boil. Like he was a child making a matter of fact statement that the sky was blue.

Pulling out two mugs, he began to put the juice of half a lemon and some slices of fresh ginger into each.

"Your body is not ready to digest a meal immediately after waking up. It needs some time to kick start the digestive fires. You can think of the lemon and ginger as kindling for the fire. The body begins to produce more enzymes with the acidity of the lemon, which brings an alkaline level to the body after absorption, and the metabolism picks up with the ginger. Add in a teaspoon of honey for the immune system and, voila, this is your morning rise and shine."

"So we're not going to eat food?" Daniel's skepticism was written all over his face even before he said anything. That look of trepidation betraying a man who had not missed a meal in a very long time.

"Drink Daniel." Looking into the mug, the wagon wheel of the lemon slice was spinning in a slow clockwise direction. One granular seed lodged into a wedge acting as the only marker to take away from the symmetry of the fruit. The pieces of ginger were bobbing and floating around the bottom of the cup. Steam was floating in wisps and dancers-like rhythm. The warmth went to his belly but seemed to radiate throughout his entire form. A three-dimensional experience. He closed his eyes and released an audible "Mmmmm…"

"And now that we've started to awaken the digestion, we're going to get into the rest of the body. Grab your mug and let's go Danny my boy."

"Where are we going?"

"Less talk, more follow."

Chapter 4(c): **Routine Practice**

"I don't have any more energy!" Sweat was dripping from the tip of his nose like water had been in his shower earlier that morning.

"If you have no more energy, then how is it possible for you to even be speaking? Quit your melodrama. Fait ta job." Daniel had a vision of an ex-lover, sat straddling him naked and aroused, chestnut hair hanging in her face, saying the same thing. His French was adequate enough to pick up the order to get to work in both instances. For the past 45-minutes Daniel had been "contortioning" his body and breathing through his mouth like a wildebeest emerging from a crocodile laden Serengeti flood plain. Of course what was a contortion to Daniel at this time was little more than a lengthening and opening of dormant muscles, and a pressing of range of motion limits of his joints.

"Breathe through your nose Daniel. Through the nostrils. Have you ever seen a person on the metro with their mouth hanging agape and their eyes completely lucid and conscious? No you haven't, because the two are inextricably linked. If you don't have the mental awareness to keep the mouth closed, then you don't have the mental clarity to be fully in this moment. The nose is for breathing, the mouth is for eating. So close your mouth and open your eyes."

And so it went. With verve and vigour Daniel would commit to the breath and posture he was in, until about 5 seconds later when the intensity of it all would have him gasping through his mouth again.

Physically and mentally the concentration demanded of him this morning was vastly different from the level he had grown accustomed. But there was such a deep and strangely familiar joy in exploring these things. A reward that he could not quite place his finger on. Forty-five minutes of pressing and pushing limits. It was all contained. There was no distraction. No outside disturbances. No urgent matters to attend to. Hell, there was not even the forty-five minutes.

There was just the body, his feelings and emotions at the moment, and of course there was…

"Through the nose Daniel!"

…the breath. For almost every posture, muscles would shake and the whole body convulse. Receiving self induced G-forces not only at the request of this man, but also from a deep river urging him to action. As though he was doing it all from and for himself.

"We work when we work and we rest when we rest. It is the only sane option. For someone to think about resting when they should be working, and thinking about working when they are in a place of rest, is not only inefficient, it's ridiculously insane."

Supine on the ground, physically full, Daniel sank into the luxury of exhaustion reserved for those who have truly put their best foot forward. Arms at his side, palms facing up, the belly moved up and then down again. Up and then down. An enchanting hypnotic rhythm. Undulating up and then down.

There is a place between the sleeping and waking state. A realm of surrender, allowance, and "no words". Where vulnerability is strength, and the intelligence of the body and creation supplies and nourishes the entire form. Within this interstice is the suspension of time and space. And with no time or space, there is a formless nature that is allowed to go beyond the normal limits and restrictions placed upon it by a mind desperate for labels and quantities. The releasing of "Who" you are and the awakening to the essence of "What" you are.

Unlike the earlier morning abrupt wake-up call, Daniel was this time ushered back into the present with a deep melodious singing. At first it seemed so subtle and distant that he couldn't exactly tell if he was hearing it, or creating it from a figment of his imagination.

"Ooooooommmmmmm…"

Each cell of his body was full, and in harmonic frequency resonating from the depths of this man's baritone.

Way back, somewhere in the distant recesses of his mind, Daniel heard a voice asking what the man's name was. The part of his brain that would have thought that to be a pertinent or important piece of information was, however, more like a wisp of dream memory. There, and then gone again, leaving with an almost imperceptible imprint.

Arising from the interstice of his practice, Daniel had a bubble of calm surrounding him. Feeling and hearing his breath like a deep-sea diver or astronaut. With that space of calm and containment, movements were slow and thoughts more viscous.

Chapter 4(d): **Routine Breakfast**

"Now Daniel, now we feast." *Funny,* Daniel thought, *I'm not even hungry.*

Walking into the kitchen, this curly haired character, ushering Daniel into place, began to pull out a bag of bulk rolled oats from the cupboard.

There are different ways of feeding and nourishing the body. Beyond that of simply ingesting something. When the signal of "hunger" is sent to the brain, it is not always the stomach that is initiating the response. Art or music. Exercise or body work. Reading or writing. Gardening or bathing. As many hobbies or activities that one can think of, one can feed oneself with these sources. To feel full, to have satisfaction, to be sated, is not always coming to people in a physical medium. Being able to distinguish and decipher the messages of the body is to be sage steward of the wants and needs of the whole system. Practicing restraint when proper, and allowing release when necessary.

Of course there is also the more conventionally preferred way to eat.

"Cup of rolled oats, cup of almond milk. Put 'em in a pot and turn on the element. Simple yes?"

"I guess so"

"Great enthusiasm Poopypants. Tell you what, go have another shower to shed the layer of your practice, and by the time you get back, breakfast shall be served."

During his quick rinse, Daniel's stomach was gurgling and doing back-flips in anticipation.

True to his word, when Daniel returned to the kitchen, a piping hot bowl of oatmeal was placed before him. To sit down now, after all the effort that he had expended in the morning hours, was to take in the vision of the steaming gruel as something close to salvation.

"There's raspberries, hulled hemp seeds, and a couple spoonfuls of real maple syrup in there as well."

"God it's delicious." Much like the hot water and lemon had warmed his insides, the heat and hearty nature of the oats seemed to settle and hug his insides.

CHAPTER: **Day to Day**

Ten past nine in the morning, 3 hours of practice in one form or another behind him, Daniel stepped out of the big red door of his apartment and into the uncertainty of the day. With the bubble of serenity still very much present, his eyes were marveling at the sights of nature and the city surrounding. This was not the same Daniel doing the same a.m. walk to the metro.

Montreal has such a myriad of different cultures. For one riding the metro it is like a United Nations on wheels. A car filled with every conceivable creed, colour, size, shape and lifestyle. Recollecting the first time he ever got on one of the rubber wheeled trains Daniel could distinctly hear 5 different languages. He loved that. He loved that there was such an admixture in the city. Of course while the historic lines of French and English being in the east and west respectively had remained relatively intact, the variety and placement of nationalities were dispersed throughout the entire city. Seemingly without rhyme or reason.

Daniel came to the hub of Montreal's underground every morning. Station Berri UQAM. The francophone tinged accents distinctly separating the sounds of the acronym, "Ooh-Cam." It is at all times, but especially during the rush hours, a beehive of activity.

It is the station at which the orange, green and yellow lines converge in order for people to get in and out of the downtown area. And like any beehive people moved with efficiency and tunnel vision.

32 e-mails, 12 phone messages, 29 texts, and 106 facebook notices. *...I really need to reset my profile settings...* Daniel had been away from his blackberry since his office dash the previous day. There was a luster and shine about him as he walked towards the metro. Walking in a slow fluid cadence, quarter past 9 in the morning, and Daniel had already lived a life since waking up.

Of all the messages that he had received, 2 e-mails and one phone call were in regards to business that he would need to attend to upon arriving at the office. The others were a variety of invitations (mostly to go drinking), random drunken messages, and a few booty calls. Please remember that this was a Monday night. Scrolling through and deleting with expert efficiency, giving quick courtesy replies to those requiring them, Daniel could hardly contain how energized he was. Trying to refrain from bursting into giggles like Ebeneezer Scrooge had done after the ghostly visits the night previous. To put it into his own words, he was feeling "fucking charged".

To wait around during morning rush hour, even ten minutes, is to watch a mass migration of ipod listening, newspaper reading, coffee drinking souls.

The entire machine moves efficiently with trains at two-minute intervals. And there is no diminishing in the number of passengers that exit and enter each one of the nine blue cars for the better part of three hours.

On average 75% of commuters would have one, if not all of the aforementioned distractions. Sprinkled in with them you have sunglasses, which is another way of shutting down or tuning out the "real" world.

Daniel was not normally in that majority. In one way or another he found entertainment in the watching or talking with others. Not to mention that when he arrived at work, with the exception of yesterday, he had to be, and was, turned on into game face mode. This little commute was an opportunity to be in the craziness of it all without the responsibility of having to control or arrange the craziness.

So while some people shut down or close off in the world of public transportation, doing so to conserve or protect energy, Daniel was actually able to recharge himself in that atmosphere. Feeling a sense of comradeship in the community of commuters.

"Hey buddy." Sticking his head around the corner of Daniel's office door, Jared was, for lack of a better description, Daniel's sidekick. "You're looking a lot better today."

"I'm feeling a lot better." An up swell of contented pride softly bloomed in Daniel's smile.

"Yeah, so what was up with you yesterday?" The comment and overall appearance of Daniel was almost completely unnoticed "I tried to phone but got the answering machine. Then I sent you a couple BBM's, and then I facebooked you."

"Oh... uh," Daniel's calm waters had just had a giant rock thrown into the middle "... nothing serious. I just had a, uh, something weighing on my mind."

"And now she's gone?" Jared's face got that slightly sneering knowing smile of a man with his mind almost permanently, in one form or another, in the gutter. If they had have been standing in close proximity, there is no doubt, he would have elbowed Daniel in the side.

"Haha," A half-hearted laugh. "Yeah, something like that." Daniel didn't exactly want to get into the specifics of a nameless man now staying in his condo.

"Well, you missed one hell of an awesome night at Cherry. The ladies were out in full force. Seriously man, like a four to one ratio." A little blip of fire went up in Daniel's mind. As though he might have missed out on something. "That girl Lindsay was there. Dude she was looking ridiculously hot dude." Another blip, this time in his belly. "She was asking about you. Seems you might have made an impression." Blip, this time more physical from the base of his genitals. Within the span of 45 seconds, Daniel's thoughts had gone from a fully focused member of the company, to a raging philistine. The gravity and pull of easy, self-satisfying desires taking him in hand.

Jared, for his part, without Daniel interrupting due to his own reveries, went on his own tirade of descriptions of what could have been, what should have been, and what actually was... almost.

Shorter than Daniel, a little heavier, with a touch less hair on his head, and a touch more hair on his neck, Jared had the remarkable male quality of thinking his chances of seduction lay within his good looks and charm. Unfortunately, where they truly were was in the fact that he was always up for a party. Up for one more drink, one more bar, one more substance. What was a precarious slope for Daniel, was an all out slip and slide for his friend. Always willing to lead the charge into debauchery and the annihilation of one more taboo. When a woman was ready to compromise a boundary of integrity due to intoxication or otherwise, Jared was there to capitalize.

Daniel was spent. The travails of his thoughts had not been particularly base, or even wholly upon the idea of the young woman, but the tug of war between where his focus and energies had stemmed from this morning, into where they had nosedived in the previous minutes, had created effort and friction.

"So what do you say?" By the time all was said and done, Jared had talked for 15 minutes.

Realizing he had barely heard anything that had been said after Jared's initial foray. "Oh, Excuse me?"

"I said did you want to come to the 5 a 7 at Philemon after work?" '5 a 7' (Pronounced "sank a set") is Montreal's version of happy hour, and an institution of when and how business gets done.

...*Yes! Yes you bastard,*... Screamed his mind. ... *Holy shit YES! That is exactly what we need. I mean I, yes I need, because I am you. You and I are one. That is to say I am I. I need to go there...*

"Uhm... I don't know if I can... I might have to head somewhere after work." *The Self shall uplift the Self; the Self shall not degrade oneself.* Whether he knew it or not, Daniel had also been repeating that through the tug of war hamster wheel battle.

"Whatever dude, I know the brush off when I get it. Just don't forget your purse when you leave Sweetie Pie." With that pearl of frat boy guilt successfully laid, Jared made his exit. Looking at his watch it was just past 11 in the morning. Daniel sat back in his chair, resting the back of his head on the cushy support, and heaved a deep sigh.

The human body is in continual homeostasis. Blood pressure, ph level, body heat, everything is within certain acclimatized boundaries. Any minor change to those levels can have profound effects to the overall organism. Another word for profound might be uncomfortable. Another word for uncomfortable could be shocking.

What this means is that the body does not distinguish between "good" change and "bad" change, it only knows that change is happening and it has to keep within its set limits. Going too far to either extreme generally means repercussions designed to retain the status quo. The potency and integrity of one's resolve is put to the test within the initial stages of change to one's lifestyle, because there is always the part of the self, whether the particular shift is a healthy one or not, that will object.

Breathing more shallow, the inrush of thoughts was a stampede of wild horses. All of which seemed VERY important. All of which clamoured to be heard and given weight. All of which would be second, third, and fourth guessed ad nauseam. The tug of war had now turned into a hamster wheel, with Daniel dutifully running faster and faster.

Chapter 2(c): Daniel History Work

For the past 6 years Daniel had worked at Amethyst Trust as a public relations liaison. The bulk of that title had him dealing with clients and prospective clients. Or as some were wont to say "Money and Big Money". It was, internally speaking, an irrelevant position for the functioning of the company. Externally, it was possibly the most influential to the overall business making its profit margins.

With that ambiguity of his necessity inside the company, Daniel was given a lot of leeway when it came to being in the office. Production was a client's happiness, and that didn't always happen from 9 to 5.

Nonetheless he made it a point to arrive just before ten in the morning, without fail as to how late he may have been out the night previous. There was none of the fanfare in how "bad" he felt in the morning. No social posturing as to the strange and odd competition of who, exactly, felt the shittiest.

It was a quality that had earned him much respect and promotion with his superiors. Engrained by childhood observance of his father, who really only seemed to be at ease when doing one form of work or another. As though through his actions he told Daniel to "Buck up. Do your job. No matter what."

So he would simply show up and take care of whatever might be in need of attention. He liked the social atmosphere and relationships bred through commonality and time. And if there was nothing pressing, well, he could do pretty much anything he pleased. For many people, Daniel included, this was a dream situation. "Do what you do, get paid for it."

Stretching in his reclined position he decided to do something about his current dispossession. Getting up from his chair with conviction, walking to his office door in a determined and powerful gait, he hung a right, walked to the end of the hall, acknowledging the few people he passed along the way, and firmly, yet quietly, stepped into the men's room to see a man about a dog.

Chapter 5: The Equation

"That, my friend, is the equation." They were in Daniel's kitchen. The countertop covered in fresh vegetables and the makings of dinner.

"The equation?"

"If you're ever uncertain or wavering in terms of a decision, you simply put it into the equation."

"Please enlighten me." Said with only slight mocking.

"Say you're in a situation that requires a decision BUT…" He held up his index finger into the air "…there are two factions within your head fighting for their own choice, and both have their own reasons behind them. Without the equation it can turn into a schizophrenic game of hopscotch, back and forth, between the two opposite ends of the spectrum. Which we'll simplify plainly by stating healthy and unhealthy."

There was little movement from Daniel. Watching him prepare the food was crisp movements linked together, with a ferocity that was deft and gentle in its handling.

"The end of that back and forth is a toss up and haggard commitment one way or the other. It opens up all sorts of uncertainty and second guessing after the fact. So even if you were to make the best decision you would continue to question your actions. Which is unhealthy and crazy all unto itself"

"It's heavy." Daniel nodded his head in a knowing gesture. His whole nervous system could recall the perpetuation of many half-hearted decisions, having relived a multitude of 'what could have been's' and 'what should have been's'.

"So THE EQUATION," enunciating those two words in a drawn out higher pitch "is this.

Anytime you find yourself in another 'This or That' circumstance, and the circumstance will be <u>ADDING</u>" He clapped his hands together "to your person, let's say the second piece of chocolate cake, buying a new sweater, watching another television show, or that drink at last call..." looking intently at Daniel and pausing for a moment "... the answer is always 'No.'"

The precision artistry of a man wielding a knife is enough to transfix anyone. Metal through colour. Daniel's breath was an almost imperceptible rhythm. The regulated clack clack clack of knife-edge to cutting board was interspersed with the sound of whatever was being spliced. The preparation of food is a delicate dance.

"When the uncertainty in deciding is dealing with," Here he started to wipe his hands. "<u>SUBTRACTING</u> something from your form, for example having a shower, exercising, going to the bathroom, drinking a glass of water... well my friend, the answer is always..." Pointing to Daniel with expectancy,

"...Yes?"

"YES! Yes Daniel!"

"But you said drinking water? And that's adding something isn't it?"

"No Smartass, it's cleansing and clarifying. The body, when dehydrated, has no end to its deficiencies. If we are 55, or 60, or 65, or 70% water like we've been hearing for however long, then the proper functioning of our systems is absolutely and unequivocally dependent upon it."

"Right. Gotcha. Never have chocolate cake or watch T.V. again." The mocking not so slight or subtle this time.

"That is not at all what I said to you Daniel. IF, IF you are uncertain. IF you're wavering as to which decision you should make, THEN you use the equation.

We're not breeding you to be a fascist dictator of your life. The problems in your life are not stemming from the instances when you are wholly committed, wholly loving, and wholly present. Some would even say that that is the purpose in life. To paraphrase Goethe, commit and providence will follow."

The two plates were beginning to take form. Each one being given equal servings of the fresh deep greens, bright red Quebec strawberries, seared almond slivers, and hulled hemp seeds. Yellowy green sunflower sprouts and crumbled goat's feta cheese, all glistening with a coating of blueberry mustard vinaigrette.

"Utilizing the equation keeps you on steady ground until you can get your bearings and wits about you again. And by not adding anything to your life, which is already confused as to what decision to make, we don't convolute an already murky decision. Where you're getting snagged is that quicksand of half-hearted actions."

Daniel thought about the bowl of soya sauce.

"And by taking something away in other situations, we'll assure that if nothing else, things might be even minutely more clear than what they were previous."

"Plus the minus. Minus the plus."

"Nice! I like that. When you're not making flaccid jokes to cover up your insecurities you have an astoundingly insightful character. You just put the whole premise into 6 words."

Daniel laughed. His hand came up to his cheek that felt the poignancy of the compliment to supercede the comment about his sense of humour.

"It's Percival by the way."

"Sorry?"

"My name. My name is Percival." It had amazed Daniel in that moment that in the three days it had been since they met, whenever they were hanging out, he had never gotten around to asking. He slightly shook his head in disbelief.

"You know it's amazing that I had yet to ask you that. There were times when it had crossed my mind, but we either got involved in something else, or I wasn't here."

"In some ways it's not all that remarkable. We've been dealing with your life. Your bubble. As you've gotten absorbed in yourself, the extraneous information like my name gets put on the back burner. And rightly so really. Worrying about stuff like that is like worrying about what colour the life jacket is when your ship is sinking."

Percival put the plates before them. The simplicity of the presentation was matched by the vibrancy and variation of the colours.

"This looks amazing."

"The preparation and care of the food is just as much part of the meal as eating the food itself." That made complete sense to Daniel but it was an odd thing to hear stated out loud. "As we say grace, I'd like you to simply look at the food before you. Let your hands rest at either side of your plate,"

Saying this, his own hands surrounded his meal as though he was holding a cat's cradle. "And allow yourself to feel this food to be specifically meant for your body. Envision the energy of your very cells to be equilibrating the frequency of the food to your own." Daniel said nothing, looking at his plate with the directions given made him feel a little silly and uncomfortable.

...Grace? Energy of my cells?...

Chapter 4(e): **Routine Grace**

"Heavenly Grace, thank you for this wonderful bounty with which you have provided before us today. May it bless, nourish, and revitalize our souls, minds, and bodies. Giving to us direction and discourse, peace, patience, and poise, and a joy of love, light, truth and understanding.

May you bless those that had a hand in bringing us this bounty today and give to them all a sense of fulfillment and enjoyment in their lives.

May you bless those that crossed our paths today. Near and far. Then and now. Who brought with them lessons, gifts and blessings, and give to them the same sense of possibility and love that you so generously and continuously bestow upon us…Amen."

"Amen." To give thanks, this would be their practice before every meal.

Chapter 6: Mind-World

Montreal is a circus town. During the summer months, one can go to any park on the island and find someone, or many people, doing an activity that makes the common man stop and watch, or cause little children to exclaim, "Mommy look!" (or "Mamam regarde!")

In that way the bustling beauty of the North American Hong Kong is at its absolute best. Free smiles, free spectacles, and generally, free lessons from the performer.

The fountains in the lake at Parc LaFontaine were at full height. Giving the area a background blanket noise to fill in the space of bird song.

They were now sat on a park bench overlooking a colourful scene. What was once two men juggling and doing the odd acrobatic move, was now a group of about a dozen people all flipping, tricking, or practicing alone or together. Feats of minor or major physical ability.

"Go back two hundred or even a hundred years ago and people were more connected to nature. They rose with the rising sun and adjusted their lives through the changing seasons. Much of what was done rotated around the earth and peoples connection to it.

Come back to the present day and practically everything within the city that you see was once a thought. Someone had to think of that lamppost or garbage can before it could ever be created. Nature does not just build an 8-storey apartment building Daniel. A city, by and large, is a reflection of the collective psyche of the culture which created it."

Watching the group swell was like watching long lost friends come together at the airport. Smiles and hugs and laughter. Daniel was an admixture of joy and envy. One heartstring being pulled regarding the free and easy playfulness, and another being struck with longing and anxiety at the thought of joining in with them. His whole stomach rumbling in a gradually increasing knot of acidic butterflies.

"So you have the population of a big city, a couple million people let's say, waking up in their rooms that were first constructed in someone's mind, to the alarm clock which records the thought construct of time. They jump into their thought car or hop on the thought bus that is traveling down the thought roads until they get to work. And what do a large portion of people do once they get to their job? They jump on this massive vortex of the mind, the computer. At the end of the work day, they commute back home, and chances are, flip on the television to get blitzed in a different form, by a world mind-obsessed and image heavy."

Daniel was transfixed. Percival's dialogue was the primary focus of his attention, and the group was intermingling with these words. As though the group's actions were one being aligned with the entire moment. Their listening was being expressed through their collectivity.

"Nature purifies the mind Daniel. It balances out the gravity of what the mind creates. Think of the awe or quietude that is formed when you are in the middle of an untouched beach along the ocean or pristine mountain range, and that's just it, there are no thoughts. That immensity of what surrounds you helps filter out the mind because it begins to feel that there is something so much more grand than it's trivial pursuits. The mind recognizes the supreme power of silence.

When people go crazy, Daniel, when they go "out of their mind", what is actually happening is that they are going wholly INTO their mind. They're not going out of their mind they're going out of their spirit. They have disassociated from the very love that they are most in need of.

Thoughts, for the most part, without action are pollution. They do nothing but wreck a perfectly good silence." With a fast smile and a quick laugh, Percival burst up from the bench and joined the barefoot revelers.

The amazing thing was how quickly and seamlessly he was absorbed by them all. Being received in a way that was not unlike how any of the others were welcomed. Never once did he glance back or beckon him to join.

Which increased Daniel wanting, absolutely, to join in as well. The riotous voices clambering about how foolish or idiotic he would look were he to go also increased their pitch. Self-aggrandizing visuals of everybody (especially the women) really liking him, polarized with the reprimand of having no skill set to offer.

That was the kicker that kept him glued to his seat. This was not a bar or a party where people were swayed by grand gestures of money or drinks. Each one of these people, Percival included, had a palpable quality about them of actually having created something with their body. And that quality was not a physical feature or attribute. It was an adaptability and way of holding space. It was an expression of their freedom in the moment.

A man walking on his hands or a pair doing acrobatic balances with one another created a sense of ineptitude and impotence. Daniel, placing himself in direct comparison with people who had conceivably spent years honing and mastering their craft, was paralyzed. That impotence stemmed from his own knowledge, conscious or not, that he had done little to nothing in comparison. He was doomed in that juxtaposition. The more he was absorbed into the harangue of belittling his self for how little had to offer, the more he would rail against this

...<humph> "teacher" who has come into OUR life and fucked everything up!...

He was not able to see the beauty of the day, the shining sun. Fresh breeze in the trees. The tranquility of lounging people reading books or children laughing chasing seagulls and squirrels, who were in turn, being chased by their parents.

The humidity in the air was enough to stick his shirt to his skin. After about half an hour he realized that he was sweating profusely.

Percival was walking back towards him. Grass-stained feet and shirtless, his entire form was proportioned and svelte. No trace of a tattoo or piercing. Daniel heard Jim Morrison and The Doors in his head "...and we laughed like soft mad children..."

"People are less connected to nature now. This, over time, anaesthetizes people. And sure anesthesia numbs people to hurtful or negative emotions, but it also blocks off the joyous and celebratory reasons for living."

"It's amazing, I've been sat here for God knows how long, and you pick up right with the same tangent you were going on before you went and traipsed about with the circus people."

"You know the saying 'Ignorance is bliss'?"

"Who doesn't? I think I heard someone say it yesterday."

"Well ignorance is not bliss. Bliss is bliss. Ignorance is anesthetic. They say that ignorance is bliss, but this is a misnomer. Ignorance is anesthetic. Ignorance is a numbing and a deadening. Ignorance is a closing down to life. And that slow choking out of any form of motivation is many things in this world, but it is definitely not blissful. It numbs you to the reality of your problems and covers up the symptoms rather than dealing with the root of the problem. Physical, mental, emotional, or psychic pain. When the level of ignorance is not sufficient to cover up the growing disease, whatever it might be, the individual comes to a crossroads. One direction is deeper into ignorance."

"Like Bret Favre."

"Excuse me?" The question was a coup for Daniel. It was the first time that he had felt like he got the drop on the ever-present Percival.

"Bret Favre. All-star quarterback in the N.F.L. He was addicted to painkillers. When a certain amount of the pills wasn't enough to kill the pain he had to up the dosage."

"That's exactly it!" The light jumped from his face when he said it.

"So I guess if one choice is to take more painkillers, the other choice is to wake the fuck up."

"Haha, the one problem with waking up though is that you have to deal with the accrued residue of ignorance that has built up over time. There's only so long you can sweep things under the bed. And that is exactly what you have been

dealing with here on this bench while I have been off..."
Here, with his elbows attached to his sides and forearms
parallel to the ground, he fluttered his fingers "...traipsing as
you put it, with Jean-Pierre, Patrick and company." Daniel
laughed a bit and realized just how much he was rolling over
in his head. He took a deep breath and looked up to the top
of the highest trees in the park. They were waving. From side
to side, painting the sky with their broad strokes. They had
been doing it the whole time.

"Let's go Daniel!" Percival, sandals in his hand, t-shirt
hanging out of the side of his shorts, was already 50 feet
away from where Daniel had been sitting all along.

"Where?!"

"Does it matter!?"

CHAPTER 7: Babysitting Dylan

The man sat opposite Daniel on the metro had a plastic Dollarama bag hanging from his wrist. Reading the business section of the English newspaper the National Post. As he turned the paper around to read the other side, Daniel read the headline of a company expecting 339$ billion in profits. Neither the man holding his recently purchased dollar store items, nor Daniel, saw the irony in the situation.

After the mental tantrum in the park, Daniel was sedate and calm. Allowing the acceleration and deceleration of the train to move him from side to side with little resistance. People got on and got off at every stop. Each person on their way to, or on their way from, a destination of import. All the while, the automated female voice declared "Prochain station..." (Next station...) to the travelers.

Being the middle of the afternoon there were not too many people getting on and off of the train. A man with a bicycle leaned against the back wall of the cab. A couple holding hands, both with sunglasses and an ear bud from the same headphones in one of their ears.

Percival leaned closer towards Daniel. He was laughing to himself in the way one does when remembering an old story.

"I was babysitting my nephew Dylan. I was 17 and he couldn't have been more than 2 or 3 years-old at the time. It was at my sister's place in the city, and Dylan was in his room. I think my sister and her husband were on a night out. Dinner and a show and all that." Daniel was intrigued by the small doorway of information being offered about this man, that he knew so little (surely not nothing?) about.

"I was watching a movie in the living room at the time" Here he paused and looked up and off into the distance. "It was Dead Poet's Society, man great movie." Daniel nodded his head. It had been a seminal movie for him in his adolescence.

"I got wondering what it was that Dylan was up to. I mean, normally he was so noisy, jumping, bouncing, asking to play. And here there hadn't been a peep for at least an hour. So I called out to him. 17 years old, man you know I didn't want to get off that couch. Call a little louder... same thing, no answer. So I got up and started walking towards his door. It had all sorts of stickers on it with no discernible pattern. As I got closer I could hear the faintest sound of Dylan talking to himself. That melodic sing-song voice when a kid is playing make believe alone." Daniel got a vision of a little boy playing legos and making up an entire civilization with a hundred or so colourful pieces.

"There was a point when I got to the doorway and had my hand on the handle that I felt like everything was,…"

"…Prochain station Villa Maria…"

Percival's ears perked up and he looked out the window. A blur of yellow, orange and red benches slowed to show 4 separate seats all a slightly different 70's shade of one of those three. The colour from each seat was extended along the ground to the platforms edge by matching coloured tiles. And each block of seats was separated from the next by about twenty or so feet.

"Let's get off here." He slapped his arm and was up in an instant to the sliding doors. They exited the front car and had the whole length of the platform to walk to the stairs and the exit. Daniel prided himself on getting on the train at the point where he would then be closest to the exit of the destination station. Getting off as far away as possible was a little burr in his saddle.

…We could have gotten on the last car at Sherbrooke…

They were halfway down the platform and everyone had already ascended the stairs on their side.

"Everything was what?"

"It's a good story so far eh?"

"Yeah, it's great. Don't play with me here. Everything was… what?"

"Well, I felt as though, with my hand on that handle, everything was exactly as it needed to be. On the outside of Dylan's little world, hearing his contented voice creating and conversing with all the characters he could imagine, that I could just go back to the living room and finish watching the movie."

"This is pretty Disney Percival. You're telling me this story because, what? Life is grand and pure?"

"Haha not quite. I opened the door… and sat in the middle of his room, diaper taken off, and happier than the proverbial pig, was Dylan." Daniel started laughing.

"And I'm not talking a little bit of shit Daniel, it was everywhere! There were handprints on the walls, designs on the floor. He was patting it when I walked in." Percival's hand gestures and mannerisms were getting more flagrant, wild, and expressive the more Daniel laughed.

"So here I am, completely dumbstruck, my hands are grabbing my hair, and my breath just drops out of my lungs. I ask Dylan 'Dylan what are you doing?' but in my head I'm yelling 'Dylan what the fuck is happening here?!' He looks up, with the sweetest face. Honestly, it was cherub-like. He has a dollop of crap on his left cheek, and as he smiled it rose up close to his eye. So I start blathering out so many questions "Why didn't you call Uncle Percival? Why didn't you leave your diaper on? We could have stopped this. I could have helped you to get changed. Why did you do this? We could have made it so you didn't have to get covered in poo."

By this time Daniel was in hysterics. The description of this little boy sat in his room, playing delightedly in his own excrement, was so comedic to him.

"So after a couple minutes of me belaboring the fact that this didn't need to happen, and that, if he had have called me we could have made it so he wasn't absolutely covered in feces, he stopped me mid-sentence with a phrase I will never forget for as long as I live. "But Uncle, I LIKE playing in my poo… I like it."

CHAPTER 7(A): Babysitting Daniel

Standing on the corner of Monkland and Girouard, the pair had come to a lovely main street kind of neighborhood with wide sidewalks and little terraces. A line of local small business cafes and shops on either side. Daniel was wiping tears from his eyes, and feeling the warmth and ache in his cheeks from the laughing.

"So what did you do?"

"What else could I do? I spent the rest of the evening giving him a bath, cleaning and disinfecting. I earned my 8$ an hour that night I'll tell you that." They both laughed into silence.

"So what was the point in telling me that story?"

"Are you hungry? I'm hungry. Let's go in this place." Percival was pointing to a little restaurant across the street with a purple awning. They walked into the Juicy Lotus needing to brush past a couple that was just exiting with their to-go.

While the woman behind the counter was dealing with the next in line she still took the split second to acknowledge Daniel and Percival with a smile and a nod. She was aglow in the hectic nature of one person after the other. Flustered, but fully enjoying that fact. Dark black hair, deep red lips, and a Mediterranean skin warm and womanly.

The glass deli counter in front of her was filled with fresh and colourful salads and sandwiches. All made that day. All in their own way tantalizing and inviting.

"So you're curious as to why I told you that story?"

"Yeah of course, I know enough about you now that there has to be some reason."

"Hi, may I help you?" They both turned in unison to be greeted by the natural smile of welcome.

"Yes please. You see before you two very hungry gentlemen." She laughed and leaned a little more heavily into her arms. "What is your special of the day?"

"Well we have your choice of salad with either soup or a wrap which is in the fridge to your right."

"Beautiful, Daniel, do you know what you'd like?"

"Uhhh…"

"That's a no then." He smiled and gave a wink to the woman. "I'll take the soup and the sweet potato salad." Daniel walked to the fridge and scanned the choices. His eyes restless and uncertain. Hearing a laugh from a couple seated by the window, he turned to see the woman bite into a burger.

"I'll have the burger please."

"And which salad?"

"Uh… The rice one."

"Perfect, broccoli kale soup and salad, and a quinoa millet burger with salad. Is that for here or to-go?"

"For here most definitely."

"Great, have a seat and I'll bring it out for you."

Bench seats of burgundy, walls of a pomegranate red, and Buddha statues adorning shelves gave the space a warm eastern motif. They took their seats flanked by others enjoying their meals and company.

"Ok my friend, so here's the reason for my little anecdote."

"I'm all ears."

"You were sat on the park bench for a long time. Brooding in whatever it was that you were obsessing about. And rather than getting out of that encompassing fog to come play with the group, you were completely contented to play in your own shit."

Daniels defensiveness immediately sprung into action.

"That's not fair! You just got up and left me!!" His voice had at least doubled in volume. Percival sat and held eye contact. All ears and eyes in the room had turned in their direction. Daniel flushed red from his outburst and started to fiddle with his napkin.

"Let's go back to Dylan. What would have happened if I got angry? What would have happened if, God forbid, I picked him up and started yelling at him?"

"He probably would have started fighting you."

Exactly. And I wouldn't just be fighting with a little boy who was, to him, just doing what was normal and natural, I would have been dealing with a little boy covered in shit."

"And I was dwelling in my own shit." He said this more with grave consternation than anything.

"That's what I love about you Daniel, you're ready and aware enough to confront yourself on aspects of your ignorance, but you're almost unrelenting in your expectation not to have any."

"So what should I be like?"

"Let me answer that question with a question. Should I get mad, I mean really get mad, at a three year-old who does something inappropriate?"

"No, of course not."

"And why not?"

"Because they don't know any better."

"Of course they don't. So what should I do?"

"Well assuming you are the child's guardian, you should parent them."

"Good, how would I do that?"

"Dependent on the situation, after rectifying the misstep, you show them a better alternative."

"Ok, would you get mad at them, I mean really mad, if instead of listening to your sage advice they threw a tantrum?"

"Well no I suppose not."

"Why not?"

"Because…uhm… I guess I wouldn't because…"

"Here you go gentlemen." She smiled as she lay down their meals, once again at ease in the service. "Would either of you like a drink?"

"…Just water please."

"Saved by the bell."

"Sorry?" She looked a little puzzled.

"Oh nothing, I'm just being a smart ass. I'll take a kombucha please."

Daniel's face went quizzical. "Come-who-ha?" This made them both burst into laughter.

"Kombucha is a probiotic tea. It's full of live cultures and millions of enzymes that eat sugars in the belly and intestines. It's great for digestion."

"Oh." He still had the quizzical look. "I think I'll stick with the water."

"Ha ha no problem. One kombucha, one water" She had told many people about kombucha to get the same response.

They sat with their meals in front of them and went through the ritual of grace. Having not eaten since that morning Daniel had been salivating for what it felt like the entire time since. Looking up from their grace, they both exchanged 'Bon appetit' and went into their own world. The next moments passing by were in silence and enjoyment, although every bite seemed to evoke from Percival a grunt or a moan after which he would close his eyes and sit back a little in his seat. Bite after bite the deliberateness of Percival was in contrast to the tenacity of Daniel.

"So the reason you don't get mad at a young child throwing a tantrum is…?"

"Because… they don't know any better." Daniel knew he had already said that.

"Let's try another tack. Would you change your guidance because of the tantrum?"

"No."

"Why not?"

"Because it's for their own good."

"Right… annnnnd?"

"And…" Daniel knew he was being led to something. He just… didn't quite… "And it's not personal!"

"Hallelujah!

"Of course. Nothing the child does is intended to hurt others. It's all about them. They're acting on self-interest, instinct and self-gratification. Even if it's at the detriment of themselves."

"And they ENJOY it Daniel. If they didn't enjoy it, they would not be in it in the first place."

"Totally."

"Exactly. Totally. There's a part of you that really loved sitting on that bench."

… *Oh fuck…* That dazed him.

"You nor I are here to get angry or judgmental at the parts of you that like to play in their own shit. What we are here for is to help that wee child to clean itself up and grow into an autonomous individual.

My not getting offended by you is not some ploy to piss you off even more. My not getting mad is because your shit has nothing to do with me."

… *Wow…* He was sinking deeper into his bench seat.

"Hell, if you can really see it, it doesn't even have anything to do with you.

Be kind to yourself Daniel. You're already emerging from the terrible twos. These next weeks are going to be some of the most expansive expressive times of your life."

He was giddy and scared shitless all at the same time within the thought of that statement. Standing at the precipice of one's own immensity tends to do that.

Chapter 8: *Twaaaaannngggg*

"Another round!!" Thursday is Montreal's Friday. Friday in Montreal is Friday squared. Thursday is a blur of businessmen urging the week to culminate. Friday is a glut of students and visiting Americans, too young to drink in their home state, desperate to grow up and experience the 18 year-old drinking limit.

Jared was in full stride. Leading the charge back to the bar, although they had never really left it.

Daniel felt powerful and thirsty for more of that surge. The foothold that they had occupied at the bar was holding a lot of gravity. Drawing attention and groups of others wanting to take part in the spectacle.

The clients whom they had earlier taken out to dinner were along for the ride. Away from their roles and home lives, it was a free ticket to self-indulgence. Beautiful tailored suits, loosened ties, and the "professional" looks beginning to fall apart at the seams.

Daniel noticed her on the dance floor. She was put together like a delicate songbird. Topped off with a 1930's detective hat. Brim pulled slightly over her eyes. She was holding off in her movements as much as she was holding off in giving her eye contact to anyone but her friends. Underneath that reserve was a supple and fluid movement. A maturity that let others know that she knew she was the prettiest girl in the room. An enigma holding back.

Philanthropy at the bar gains anyone a wealth of bff's. There's something so very invigorating in having the thrust and flow of the nightclub trying to get closer to you. A corset of penny pinching hands giving support. Jared was clutching right back. Garish comments and sincere laughter urging his compatriots onwards.

"Dude, I love my life!!" Jared was 100% sincere in his statement.

"I know you do buddy." Daniel was laughing and returned the arm over the shoulder that Jared had just wrapped around his own.

"I've been worried about you dude. The past week you've been acting pretty weird." Daniel had already drank so much of the social lubricant that he was right in line with Jared's assessment of his situation.

"I completely agree with you!"

"Good." Jared was completely unsurprised to have that response. To him it was as plain as day. "Hey you want to know what else?" His grip around Daniel's shoulder got a little tighter.

"What's that?"

"Breasts are the Big Mac of our generation." Daniel started laughing. For some reason he was not at all surprised by Jared's tangent. "Think about it. The commercials you see for the Big Mac are perfect. Crisp lettuce, perfectly melted cheese, with a sizzling patty, I mean, fuck, even the seeds are placed perfectly. And then what happens when you get a Big Mac and open up the box? It definitely doesn't look the same. Lettuce is wilted and barely green, the bun is squished, there's sauce all over the place.

So now look at that girl over there. Her cleavage is on display. She's advertising the perfect Big Mac. Push-up bra and revealing top makes everything look a little more perky.

A little more round and succulent. And I am definitely sold! I am hungry for her Big Mac dude." His voice turned into a low comedic growl there. "But I'm not kidding myself. I know that what she is advertising is not exactly what's on the billboard. They're going to be droopier. They're going to have conspicuous hairs. I mean, fuck, nipples are a complete crap shoot…"

"I get it man."

"No, no, let me finish. There's one place the Big Mac and women's tits, really deliver. The taste. The TASTE DANIEL!" Daniel was almost in a complete headlock now. Jared was yelling and proclaiming like a plump, toga wearing, roman senator. That drunken reverie where the truth is so plain it deserves to be shared overtly and freely to anyone and everyone in proximity. "I'm hungry. I'm hungry for love!… Aaaaand another drink. Christ I'm thirsty. Cristophe!" The beckoning hand of nobility followed by the lean in to place the order. "Another Jack and Coke, and my friend'll have…"

Daniel had already walked away. The pull of his mystery woman had grown too strong. He walked onto the dance floor and started a generic side to side movement with the music. Her delicate jaw line was even more noticeable with it being sandwiched between the hat and a pink sheer scarf.

The moment happened when they started moving in synch for two or three beats. She looked up under the brim of her fedora and made eye contact with Daniel. Fiery eyes that were accustomed to being avoided, were held here by a firm and welcoming gaze.

After about 4 seconds she bowed her head. A demure and mischievous smile did not go unnoticed by Daniel. For the next minute they continued their subtle dance in unison. Suddenly and somewhat violently she started to push any guy that was within shoving distance with a flawless two-armed technique.

…She's trying to prove her dominance and untouchability…

In quick succession one, two, and three slightly bewildered guys received the shove off. Daniel walked straight up to her.

"Can I buy you a drink?" Without missing a beat she turned on her heels, grabbed his right hand and led them off the dance floor to the bar.

"Two tequilas!" There was a hint of a French accent as she shouted out the order. They both turned and looked at each other.

"My name is Daniel."

"Melanie" The inflection in the last two syllables was definitely francophone. Two shots were placed at their hands on the bar, which were separated by a few inches.

"Cheers!" He made eye contact again. Sharp green eyes were dangerously framed with high cheekbones.

"Santé" This was not a normal seductive look. Her serpentine eyes hypnotized Daniel as her left hand moved up to her mouth and velvet tongue purposefully lapped up the salt.

…Wow…

"I have to go to the bathroom."

"Thank you so much Melanie, it was a pleasure to meet you." Daniel was genuine in his thanks. He thought there was more, but he also didn't want to press the issue. She leaned forward a little closer and touched his forearm.

"You can be here when I get back if you'd like." She was gone before he could get as much as an "Ok" out of his mouth. His chest began to swell as he stayed completely immobile. Part of him wanted to be exactly as he was when she returned. A few minutes passed. Then a few more. He was just beginning to think that maybe he had been given an unceremonious shove-off himself, when a hand was placed on his low back and she stepped around in front of him.

"I'm glad you're back." She smiled and once again gave a slight bow of the head to the compliment. "Would you like another drink?"

"I'll have what you're having."

"Two Stellas." It's easy to be cool in the initial stages of attraction. Every movement has substance and support. Daniel's were made as though he already had everything he could ever dream. When they got their drinks she once again took his hand and led him away. This time they were circling the dance floor. Instead of their joined hands trailing low behind her, they were above her shoulder with her elbow pointed up into the air.

...She's showing me off...

There was no resistance from Daniel. In fact there was that stupid grin which was a less subtle male equivalent to being complimented.

She strode through the crowd with strength and purpose. As they almost completed a full circumnavigation she made a sharp left onto the dance floor. Straight into the densest part of the crowd. As soon as she turned to face Daniel they were deep into a pressed embrace. Hips to hips, belly to belly. Her face nuzzled into the crook of his neck. With both arms draped over his shoulders, he could feel the cold wetness of her beer bottle between his shoulder blades. His hands were exploring the smooth firm contours of her ass. Squeezing and pulling her towards him with thrusts in unison to the music. A grinding back and forth, up and down, all around movement. The world had shrunk to 2 foot square. The temperature and humidity was dense and rich.

Daniel could feel her breath creating a film of condensation on his neck. They were not just dancing with their hips and bodies, but with the pressure and placement of their heads as well. Rolling into position like wrestlers trying to get the upper hand. Cat and mouse, trading off the roles.

The closest they came to kissing was the creases of their lips brushing. Her mouth slightly open so he could feel the breath on his cheek. Her smell was light but decadent. Flowery with a hint of fruit and citrus.

As quickly as they had walked onto the dance floor, she peeled his hand off her backside and led them straight towards the three girls she had come with. The next thirty minutes was a blur of her friends talking about how wonderful Melanie was, and a series of belittling and rather aggressive comments directed towards Daniel. All of which were taken in stride with a smile and a playful self-deprecating comment.

There was no question that Melanie was good enough for Daniel, her friends were testing out whether the inverse was true.

Chapter 8(a): The Reverberation

Her key slid into the lock and they ascended the stairs to her 3rd floor apartment. The rows of houses in Montreal are traditionally fronted with spiral staircases leading up to a second floor balcony. With one or two doors that lead into the 2nd floor flats, and with one or two other doors with stairways behind, leading up to the spaces above.

Daniel, once again, and with myriad reasons, was wary of introducing anyone to his home and houseguest.

The amount of shoes in the stairwell, and then walking into the apartment, was astounding.

"You said you live alone didn't you?"

"Yes, why?" She was genuinely perplexed by the comment.

"Oh, no reason." He smiled at her and nudged a pair of pumps to the side with his feet.

"Have a seat." She walked down the hallway and gestured to her left as she kept walking and stepped into a room to the right.

Daniel walked into the living room and pushed aside a bundle of clothes off the couch to clear some space.

She was definitely an artist. Rows of canvases leaning against the wall. A select few actually hanging up. Magazines, clothing, glasses and plates, art supplies, old to-go containers, newspapers, and any host of random trinkets were strewn about without discretion.

"Is this a 5 ½?" Montreal has an odd designation for the size of apartments. A 3 ½ is a one-bedroom, 4 ½ a two bedroom, and so on.

"Yes." She walked around the corner as she said this. She had changed into a t-shirt and let her hair down. As she leaned against the doorframe Daniel stood up and walked towards her. He had resisted the attraction to kiss Melanie all night with the concept of wanting to appear in control. They locked into an embrace and sealed lips together. Her dainty tongue dancing with his. The soft clicking and smacking of saliva were the only sounds to be heard.

Daniel loved everything about this. Crossing a boundary of intimacy to discover new, fresh, and unknown movements. A stranger, for all intents and purposes, opening herself up because of a mélange of want, lust and trust.

The intensity grew as their breath grew more erratic and hands more frantically explored the other. Daniel used the leverage of his weight to press Melanie's back up against the wall. His gradually inflaming groin pulsing and pressing up against her in suggestive rhythm.

She pushed him hard away. Not unlike she was wont to do in the nightclub earlier. He stood back and smiled at her. They both took a breath. Giving a wry look and biting her lower lip she opened up her right hand to reveal two small pills in her palm.

"Do you want?" Her French accent cutting off the question halfway. Daniel immediately felt a restriction just below his sternum. That apprehension transferred to his face. While Daniel would consume copious amounts of alcohol during the week, drugs and narcotics had never really grabbed him as a worthwhile pursuit.

His mind spun calculating multiple permutations as to what to do. Looking in her eyes, he saw for the first time a fatigue that was deep, deeper than a need for sleep. She was needing something. That neediness pressed a button to his own place of fear and losing that he was unable or unwilling to enter.

"Uhm, no thanks. I'm fine right now." He had no real idea what he was saying no to.

There was a split second of hesitation on her part, as though for the briefest of instants wondering why she wanted to take the pills in the first place, and then deftly popped both of them into her mouth.

Chapter 9: Gravity of the Routine

His key slid into the lock of the red door and he stepped across the threshold of his condo. It was 5:30am and the sun had already crested the horizon to give a clear quiet light.

There is something so restful in coming home after a night out. A deep sensation of decompression and quietude.

Unburdening himself of practically everything that had been with him during the night, he walked topless into the kitchen to the surprising, but not really, sight of Percival pouring steaming hot water into two mugs.

"Good man. Here's your hot water and lemon, triple-S and I'll see you in the living room in 15 minutes."

"Good morning to you too." Daniel was surprised, but not really, at how relieved he was to see Percival, and feel like everything was still in full stride.

There was a new exuberance in Daniel's actions that morning. It was a liveliness that Percival pressed to its limits. Sensing a willing participant meant that everyone was going in the same direction. Daniel felt as though his whole form was equilibrating to one uniform viscosity. Like T-1000 from the second Terminator. His body was getting more fluid and supple as he felt his breath getting more thick and palpable.

Allowing Percival's voice to be the primary focus of his integrating mind, there was no questioning as to what he was doing or where he was being led, only a deep and full watching. Disassociated but not distant.

In a physical sense his body was only slightly more flexible than when all of this started over a week ago. The big change was in his breath. The restriction of his joints and muscles were not so tentative to accept the expansion of the lungs. Creating a snowballing effect. The larger he inhaled, that gave more space to exhale and purge the lungs. That emptying contraction led to an inhalation that was so enjoyable it was as though he was bursting out of water.

Sweat dripping into a pool beneath him, the body was, to him, running clean. Over and over he would press to a level of effort and focus that would shake the very foundation of his nervous system. And just when he felt as though he could not survive the intensity he would be verbally released from the bonds of the posture, to receive a flood of endorphins and decompression from the parasympathetic nervous system.

The stench of liquor emanating was amusing to Percival. It was all part of the process.

"One of the most important things you can learn from our time together is work when you work and rest when you rest." Daniel was lying prone on the ground. Left cheek to the earth, arms at his sides with the palms facing up. The rise and fall of his stomach against the ground was heavy and so enjoyable. "You get into an intense posture here Daniel and suddenly all you're thinking about is getting out of it. And when you get to a place of rest and absorption all you do is anticipate about what posture is next. That's not helping anything Daniel."

He was a gelatinous blob on the ground. A happy-to-do-nothing mass. A jellyfish washed up on the beach that kids poke with a stick.

"Good, rise your legs off the ground, raise your arms like airplane wings and come into full flight." The muscular shaking was slow and manageable. "Shoulders from the ears, squeeze the knees together, and get your ribcage off the ground." The shaking was now akin to the space shuttle re-entering earth's orbit. "Use it up Daniel," …*Oh god…* "5 more seconds," … *I can't do it…* "4 more," …*I'm gonna fucking die!…* "3," … *I can do this…* "Holding for two," … *I can't do this…* "Best part 1," …*Ahhhhhhhhhhhh…* "And releasing down." Collapse, blob-mode.

"The energy that you have right now is meant to be used right now. This energy is the most up-to-date technology that the body can use for its performance. And as soon as that technology is processed and used up, newer, more advanced technology comes along. Your abacus becomes a calculator. It's why you need to use it right now. A Nintendo is great, but if you're trying to get onto the internet it is completely useless.

So when you empty your cup of the energy available to you in this instant, it opens up more space for the body to refine and synthesize a more potent product. Version 2.0 ad infinitum."

Daniel wasn't even really listening. The pulse and pump of his heart, the sweaty humid lump of his body, the hiss of his breath, were all muffling Percival's speech into a Charlie Brown Teacher's tuba.

The Pixie's "Where is my mind?" would be an apt soundtrack.

… Where is my mind? Where is my mind?…

CHAPTER 10: Shit meet Fan, Fan let me introduce Shit.

"Who cares?!"

"I know right?!"

"Oh my God. Totally, so I said to her…" Daniel was standing on the metro besides two women deep in their gossip of he said, she said. The equivalent to this type of conversation in the physical world is refined white sugar. Daniel enjoyed the valley girl dialogue. A series of "likes", "ya knows", and "oh my god totallys". He was so relaxed he could have heard music in a band saw.

It was 9:32am, and on exactly zero hours of sleep Daniel could not remember the last time he felt so good going into work. He couldn't actually think of a time where he felt this good going anywhere.

"What are you looking at?" One of the women was looking at Daniel with a disgusted air. It completely knocked him out of his reverie.

"… Excuse me?"

"Were you looking at my tits?"

"Oh my god, you're, like, disgusting." Her friend chimed in immediately. Daniel was still staggering to find his footing from the initial volley.

"Uh… no I wasn't…" He was of course. It's natural for a man's eyes to gravitate towards a woman's chest when the mind is blank. It's probably some touchstone instinct from infancy. From his standpoint there was no objectification in his thoughts.

Before he knew it, in the span of the time it takes the train to get from Place Des Arts metro to McGill, he had been called any number of insults and expletives. The women's faces, noses wrinkling, upper lips raising in a half Elvis snarl, eyes lowered, looked as though they had just smelled a ripe fart. You know, fart-smelling face.

It turned into the uncomfortable public spectacle where everyone was listening but averting their eyes at the same time. The energetic version of a train wreck.

Daniel stepped out onto the platform to one final desultory "Pig" and felt his heart in his stomach. The whole situation had blown up in his face and left him covered in ugliness as he walked towards his office.

Rene Levesque is a wide boulevard along the south side of downtown. On either side skyscrapers create a chasm to frame the sky and open air above the street. The Old Port just to the south and Mont-Royal and the Plateau/Mile-End district to the north.

Silhouettes of the buildings were particularly accentuated by a crisp and brilliant light blue. Not a cloud to be seen.

For himself, Daniel was still playing over the scenario with the two women. The initial shock had turned into fantasies of what he could have said to gain the upper hand. All them biting and witty, and strangely, giving his own expression a look of fart-smelling face.

… *I was looking at your chest because you put them on display like baked goods…*

As soon as he walked into the office he stowed the event away and answered all of the small talk questions with "Fine." And "I'm good thanks, how are you?" The expressive muscles of his forehead working to feign happiness and ease.

"Shaughnessy,... Can I see you for a second please." Richard Lepage was the director of Amethyst Trust. The hanging silence between his name and the request for a meeting did not bode well for Daniel. The ugliness in his belly had grown and deepened in density.

There is nothing quite so corrosive as the feeling of an impending scolding. Especially a scolding for which you have no idea why you might even be getting reprimanded in the first place.

All he wanted from the first moment of entering the building was to get behind the closed door of his office.

Instead the door of Dicky Lepage's was shutting him in, and a normally jovial and fatherly demeanor was replaced with a cold supervisory direction.

"Have a seat Daniel." Daniel took his place with the mask of the placating 'Sure, sure thing, anything you say, no problem' attitude. "You mind telling me what happened last night?" Any question was going to take Daniel off guard. His whole body seemed to be tender and nauseous.

"Last night?" He was having flashbacks of being confronted by his Dad as a 15 year-old. "Well, uhm, Jared and I took the execs from DeNair Construction for dinner at Le Gros Jambon in the Old Port, and then we went to a couple nightclubs where we ended up on St. Laurent"

"And you were with them the whole time?"

...*Oh fuck*...

"Well I left the club at about 2."

"And where did the execs go at this time?"

"They stayed at the bar."

"You left them there alone?"

…Where is he going with this?...

"Uh, at the time no. They were still with Jared."

"That's funny, because Jared said that he had left them in your care."

…He's lying!...

"You know GOD DAMN WELL that since the get-go our policy has been to see clients back to their hotels! NO MATTER WHAT!"

…I don't think Dicky has ever yelled…

"So now I get a call this morning at 4am from one of them using his one phone call saying he needs to be bailed out."

…Holy shit…

"And not just on some drunk and disorderly charge, but on possession." Daniel's face went from dumbstruck to ashen white. "And they say they were given it by you"

…They're lying…

"Given what?" His question went unanswered.

"Think of how this looks to me Daniel. All three of your companions have directly said you were the source. And in having known you for the past 6 years I can honestly say I have never been more shocked, surprised and saddened."

"But I haven't done anything! I walked out of the bar with a young woman just after two."

"Well until this gets sorted out, you're going to have to pack your things up and vacate the premises."

"C'mon Dick, you're not serious are you?"

"You're fucking right I'm serious!" The vein bulging on the left side of his head extended from his hairline to his shirt collar. Daniel was completely unversed in confrontation like this. He knew he had to defend himself, but he had no idea where to begin with the false accusations. "I've stayed out of your affairs and been extremely lenient with how you treated our clients, but if this is how you've been getting results then you've put everything at risk."

"Dick I have no idea what you're talking about."

"I've contacted our lawyers and they've said that this is the least I need to do to protect the company." Nothing that Daniel was saying was even remotely being registered by LePage. The dye had already been cast. "Get a lawyer Daniel. That's the best advice I can give you. As of right now you are no longer under the protective umbrella of Amethyst Trust."

"Jesus Dick you can't be serious?!"

"This is the most serious I have ever been. The high school shit you pulled last night has completely broken my trust in you. I thought you were better than this."

… I am better… Better than what?…

"Dick what are you talking about? You still haven't said what I've been accused of."

"I can't stand this acting dumb routine Daniel, I'd respect you a lot more if you just acknowledged giving them the coke."

…What?!…

"What?!"

… That's not true!…

"That's not true! I've never touched that stuff in my life."

"Well if that's the case then I feel sorry for you, but right now there's a number of people all saying you're responsible and there's no reason for me not to believe them. Especially with the talk that's been happening in the past week about your strangeness."

"You're saying that in all the time of me working here you don't know that I would never do something like that?"

"Who knows anything about anyone anymore." This was a mid-sixties man talking in a generational sense now. A man who had seen the shifts of technology and societal norms pressed well beyond boundaries he once thought already too liberal. "We've all got skeletons in the closet and it looks like yours just got exposed. Who knows, maybe all this time you've been making it into the office from your late night escapades because you've been high as a kite?" The last sentence was stated more as though he had just thought of it in that moment.

Whatever it was that Daniel had had exposed, it felt as though his heart was making its way through a cheese grater. The clench of his jaw was starting to give him a headache. Withholding with every ounce of his being and character the desire to start yelling bloody murder at the injustice being perpetrated upon him. The weight bearing down and the anxiety pushing up was reaching redline proportions.

It is in this sort of catastrophic event that people collapse into a nervous breakdown. Like a computer's circuit board being overloaded with a surge of electricity and completely burning out. It gets to a point where it is the only way to handle the stress.

Massive amounts of thoughts were getting bottlenecked in his brain. Cramming like pigs at a trough in a Japanese subway car on 'Ride the subway for free day' during the Olympics.

...Am I having a stroke?...

"Daniel, I have a meeting in 10 minutes that I have to get to. I'll have security escort you off the premises." Six years of loyal and dedicated service doesn't get you what it used to. The not so subtle good-bye was the kicker.

...It's not true, it's not true, it's not true...

CHAPTER 11: **Biblical Emotions**

"Not the most inspiring mantra there is it bud?"

Percival had been listening intently to Daniel's rant for the better part of an hour. It was a comprehensive rendering because the details were still very much fresh in his head.

All the ins and outs of dinner and clubs the night previous. The courtship and connection with the beautiful Melanie, leading to how nothing happened. She had drifted off into the deeper waters of her chemical high. Daniel leaving her apartment after carrying her to bed and making her comfortable snuggled under her duvet. It was the one point of his telling that he seemed to embody in a reminiscent way.

Leading to all the frenzied proclamations towards the two indignant women in the metro who had summarily chastised and ridiculed him.

It was a fantastic story. The heaviness of the exit from the office flanked by rent-a-cops, under the watchful eyes of half his former colleagues, while the other half avoided the scene by burying their heads in their computers. There was no rocking of an already shaky ship in this office. No dramatic Jerry Maguire event was forthcoming. Daniel made no speech, and no one stood up to defend him.

There was a lot of force and fire in everything he said, but when it got to the part about the exchange in Richard LePage's office he got choked up.

It was true that the elder statesman had not intervened in his work very much, but he had thought that was more due to a mutual respect and acknowledgement of his abilities and dedication. To be unceremoniously dumped was devastating to a place inside of him that felt more closely akin to the loss of a loved one. That feeling of loss could have been the reason that he left the office and building with little more than a whimper. Only a fool rails against the dead.

Realizing that this "family", as Dick was wont to say at every staff event, was false and gone to him. That had created a void he was unable to even grasp as to how he would fill it. And physically numb to the idea of going forward.

… *It's not true, it's not true, it's not true*…

"That's a wonderful story. What an adventure!" Percival leaned back in his chair and clasped his hands behind his head.

"Story?! This is my Life!!"

"Yes, yes very dramatic. Unnecessary, but dramatic."

Daniel glared at Percival with menace and aggression. It was his intention in that moment to intimidate the smugness out of his face. To bully his way to some form of satisfaction much in the same way he had felt victimized. They stared at one another, neither one saying anything for 30 seconds. For a minute, and then two. They stared well beyond the normal confines of convention.

For Percival it was a chance to share and listen. A time to allow the moment to speak for both of them. Silence is a place where much is told, and the reflection of another's eyes offers much.

For Daniel, what started out as an act of force and will had begun to transcend into an abstract quality of seeing Percival but also seeing the Percival that was behind the face of Percival. It was a gaze of such tender and luminous love.

His light blue eyes were the only things in focus. Everything else had taken on an otherworldly dream quality, fuzzy and morphing.

The phrase "Don't stare it's rude." much like the phrase "Ignorance is bliss." is a red herring to keep people resigned to their ignorance. It's a collusion of the lazy. The directive that staring at people is impolite is designed to prevent those who have not done their interior work from being discovered. Think of it like this. Most people, with their home in complete disarray, would be embarrassed to have someone see the shambles. If nothing else, they would not invite anyone over. The eyes being the window of the soul gives others a direct viewing of all the unwashed dishes, dirty laundry and overflowing garbage cans. Likewise, one can see into a soul well cared for, fresh and clean. But of course those people are proud of their homes and are normally welcoming to others.

Holding eye contact without speaking for any length of time taps into a different sensation of consciousness. It is two consciousnesses regarding one another. It is a space which the unprepared almost automatically shatter with words or looking away.

Daniel's prideful aggression had brought him into a depth where he could not look away from Percival, and the layers he was witnessing kept his voice mute. As much as he saw love, there was also a strength and warrior nature. Old man, and young child. Fierce fighter grizzled and battle worn.

"Let's cut right to the chase." It was Percival who broke the stalemate. "Were you absolutely, 100%, living the full extent of your purpose with this last job?"

"Well no but…"

"So then it is irrelevant whether the circumstances are true or fair because, in point of fact, they have liberated you to pursue what it is that will ultimately fulfill you."

"Well no but…"

"Maybe it stings a little bit more that it happened so fast and you were on the receiving end of the break-up. Sometimes it's nice to know that we took the jump consciously, however!" He held up his index finger "we both know you were suffocating in that environment."

"Well no but…"

"And you'll forgive me for saying this" a huge smile broke across his face "I could not have planned this out better myself."

… He's laughing at us. Laughing at our pain…

"What does that mean? You're happy this happened?!"

"Happy is not the right word."

"Well what is?"

"I'd say more like, I see the perfection in the unfolding."

"You see the perfection in me being implicated as a drug dealer?!"

"Did you do it?"

"NO!!!"

"Well then what's the problem?"

"I lost my job, I lost my friends, I lost MY LIFE!"

"Yes, yes very dramatic. Let's look at those three. You lost a job that was not going to enable the growth of your Self into the man you wish to be, or even, for that matter, worthy of the man that you are."

Punch in the gut.

"Any friend that would sell you out at the first sign of collapse is not a friend, that's a tourist."

Slap in the face.

"And the life that you supposedly have lost Daniel? Your life was the straw house that the first little pig built.

Kick in the groin.

"FUCK YOU!"

"Ha ha, no Daniel, fuck you."

At this point, all of the rage, indignation, frustration, hurt, whininess, and whatever other jambalaya emotion was being repressed by Daniel let loose in a flooding spew of yell. A shrieking hissy fit of tantrum. A shit-slinging storm of fury.

Spittles of saliva flew off his lips with consonants and a gargling base of phlegm rose and fell in his throat through the vowels. Fists, neck and asshole were welded tight. Testicles sealed up against the pubic bone. There was absolutely, positively, not even the remotest inclination towards political correctness. On the contrary, he wanted to insult everyone. This was road rage in the comfort of his kitchen with no unfortunate bystanders or lookers-on. Making up words with whatever seemed available to his high blood pressure resources.

Giving the necessary "Yeah man" or "Fucking rights" at intervals to fuel the fire, Percival was right on board with the rant. Nothing quite keeps a tirade going like someone agreeing with you. He loved someone breaking down the boundaries of 'normal' and 'polite' behavior.

Atrophy is something that happens to life when life, for long enough, goes unused. And just like a business that doesn't get used goes bankrupt, a muscle unused withers, or an engine that doesn't get used rusts and seizes up, our emotions, when suppressed due to convention or societal constraint, due to an unwillingness or inability to feel them, or even due to a lack of time, will create not only a diminished ability to experience emotions, it will create a diminished ability to express emotions.

An unrestrained rant is better than having that shit fester and stagnate. And there is something ultra real about someone losing their shit. The eruptions are so flagrantly over the top that no one present would think for a second that they were responsible for the outrage. Instead one can just watch and marvel at the big hairy biblical floods bursting forth, without feeling that they were the ones responsible for the onslaught. Sort of like watching a building demolition. (Sidenote: If the person watching the breakdown has a bunch of similar shit yet to be resolved, the outburst will actually make them extremely uncomfortable.)

In the blindness of his emotions he had not noticed Percival laughing hysterically for the better part of two minutes. Tears reeling down his face and the gasping breathlessness of genuine laughter.

"What the fuck are you laughing at you fucking fuck!?" Swearing and cursing in today's culture means so much it means nothing. The versatility of profanities can be used as noun, verb, adverb, adjective, pronoun. Many people, especially when agitated, will use swear words as a default to actual articulate phrasing. The mind moving too fast to care simply belches out the easy filthy option. To put it bluntly, it's like farting out of one's face.

Wiping tears from his eyes and restraining his breath enough to get a sentence out, Percival was barely able to get out "You just said poopy anal farts…" before bursting back into uncontrollable laughter.

"No I didn't… Did I?" Daniel started chuckling to himself when he realized that he was about to argue whether or not he had actually said poopy anal farts. It was that split second that created enough space to snap him out of his tirade.

Chapter 12: **Where to Begin?**

"What kind of a name is Percival anyway?"

"My dad loved the Knights of the Round Table. In a way I think he was hoping I would emulate The Grail Legend with my life." Daniel didn't quite know what he meant.

"What do you mean?"

"One was only granted one opportunity, one chance, to attain the Grail. In the story of Percival he failed in his moment of truth. When in presence of the ailing Grail King he failed to ask him two questions."

"What were the questions?"

"'Lord, what ails thee?' was the first, and 'Whom does the Grail serve?' was the second. By not asking these questions he had fallen at the final hurdle. The idea being that only one who is pure of heart would be worthy of such a prize. If one were to already have had prior knowledge of the act, that person could hardly be considered to have the acme of purity right?" Daniel nodded at the prompt. "He awoke in the morning to find that the castle that was just the night before filled with life and majesty, to be barren and deserted."

"That's it?! Just because he didn't ask a couple questions?"

"Yup."

"But what are a couple questions going to accomplish?"

"Daniel, when the right questions are asked it's the Soul itself that answers."

… Wow… His breath froze in the statement of one awed by a response.

"So… So what did he do?"

"He began his quest again. He did not agree or believe in the verdict being rendered in stone. His commitment and earnestness had been redoubled by his failure. And though there was no hope, think about that, literally, what kind of hope can one have if it is God himself who has passed judgment? With no hope, he pledged himself once more into the quest."

"But he was just at the end. Where did he start? How did he start?"

Percival smiled. "He started where he was. He started with nothing."

The moment hung in silence. Somewhere in his head there was a dark fortress under siege. A tempest of shouts and derogatory insults lobbed from behind its battlements. Poisonous fire desperately trying to deflect the persistent and unrelenting encroachment of light.

"Until he got the Hollywood fairytale ending I suppose." The sarcasm came thick with his words.

"It has nothing to do with the end Daniel!" Percival had that blaze in his eyes. "In fact that's exactly why he ultimately changed God's will.

Your actions have been attached to some goal of satisfaction. To the idea that some THING, or some PLACE, or some ONE is going to, all of the sudden, make your life complete. You fool. You clown. You buffoon." The last three insults were levied with the same scorn and derision as the kind emanating from Daniel's rant only minutes before. But these had the effect of absolutely gutting his will in the fight. It was a dagger to his black heart. The word "clown" echoing in his head.

"This is not a time for rebuttals Daniel. This is the next step. Impossible without the one's previously taken and ABSOLUTELY necessary for the one after to present itself. Your wavering faith, while perhaps not the direct cause of your lot right now, is definitely culpable in keeping you mired in it.

Sir Percival was devoid of all hope at his rejection. His whole life had been dedicated to that one goal, and he failed. His was the biggest loss any of us can imagine. In his own ignorance he had rejected God, and his reward for such ignominy was that God in turn rejected him." Daniel's head was draped between his shoulders like a ripe piece of fruit.

"So what did he do?" His voice was a whisper. This was a voice calling from the heart of darkness. A hand reaching for some, for any, grace.

And from that question came one shard of light to pierce into the valley of the dark night of the soul.

"He chose." This simple statement, at this exact moment, in perfect divine alignment, was the truth to unshackle the bonds of his ignorance. Amazing grace, how sweet thy sound. That saved a wretch, a clown, like me.

Chapter 13: **Purging**

For the second time in just over a week, Daniel cried. Where the first time was a catharsis coming in huge bellowing wails, this second time was dirtier. There was a mucky film to his sobs. Gut wrenching, torturous, and mournful.

"What the fuck is wrong with me?" Externalized, the question was asked to himself as much as anyone. The more he felt like he was crazy or stupid for being so hysterical, the more raw and tender his entire body would become. As a grown man he was repulsed by his weakness. Basically he was sickened at being so sickened.

"What were you praying for before I got here Daniel?" Caught off guard, he just lifted his head with a quizzical look. "Do you need me to repeat the question?"

"No… I just… I…" His mind went to his times of quiet desperation. "I guess I was praying for a salvation."

"Have you found it?"

"No."

"What did you think it was going to be?"

"I don't know."

"So how do you know you haven't found it?"

"Because it shouldn't be this hard."

"Compared to what?"

"I don't know."

"Exactly."

"What does that mean?"

"How can you think that something isn't the way it should be if you don't even know what the something is?"

Daniel wanted to say 'I don't know' again, but decided to keep his mouth shut. "Denying what is, inflames it, which makes it even more difficult."

"I can understand that."

"When we pray it's like asking to increase our spiritual strength. Life gives us the dumbbells in the form of challenges for us to flex our spiritual muscle. You must have been praying pretty hard to get these weights." Daniel gave a scoffing laugh as if to say 'Yeah no shit.'

"So if you were praying for salvation, why aren't you celebrating the opportunities presented to you?"

"Because I'm scared." With his head still between his shoulders, the late afternoon sun was beginning to shine through the window. Percival leaned back on his stool and took his hands off the counter. "I'm 31 years-old and I have no idea what I'm doing."

"And how does that make you feel?"

"Scared! It makes me feel scared."

"Where?"

"In my heart. In my guts. In my skin."

"And what does it feel like?"

"Helpless. Like I'm drowning."

"And that surprises you?!" His question was given in mock surprise as though Daniel should have known better.

"What?"

"You've been damning up, diverting, or repressing your emotions for God only knows how long, and you're shocked and surprised by the power of the current?"

"But I didn't know."

"Not knowing about something is no excuse not to know about it."

"That makes absolutely no sense."

"Daniel do you remember when we first met and you asked me why I was talking about life as a sentient entity?"

"Yeah, you never really explained that to me."

"If we went to the ocean, and I started swimming into a rip tide would that current pull me out to sea?"

"Yeah of course."

"OK, what if it was my birthday or Christmas? Or what if I was two years-old and didn't know about the immensity of its power?"

"So you're saying that my actions, whether they were conscious or not, are solely my responsibility? Life does what it does, just like water does what it does."

"Bingo."

"And just because I've been ignoring my emotions is no excuse for being overwhelmed by them."

"Go on."

"I've jumped in at the deep end and now I've got to sink or swim."

"More like you created the deep end." They both chuckled at this. He was feeling more buoyant in his attitude.

"Touché."

"Look at it like this Daniel, you need to learn how to swim, and the best way to teach you is through the repetition of small important things. Saying that you don't know how to swim is a giant lead weight preventing you from learning."

"It's a burden."

"You took the words right out of my mouth. You just said you're scared and don't know where to start." Daniel felt a hot flash of multiple emotions at the thought of his plight. "Well who cares where you are if you're going to drown? You could be in the middle of the Atlantic Ocean or in the neighbour's kiddie pool but if you can't keep your head above water, where you are is completely irrelevant."

"Understood."

"Good man. You're farther along than you know Daniel... much farther." The compliment, at this time was much needed by Daniel. "Your next step is to fully commit to this salvation you've been asking for."

"How do I do that?"

"Think about the kind of man you want to be and sum it up in one sentence."

"Uhhh..." His eyes were wide with the challenge of fitting all that in sentence.

"Sleep on it man. Once again you've had a hard and huge emotional roller coaster day. The next first steps commence tomorrow."

There was little to no resistance from Daniel at this prompt. Fatigue was in his bones. Getting into bed when you don't know how tired you are is a salvation all unto itself. His bed turned into the warm cinnamon bun of sheets, duvet and body heat. All of that support bringing his nervous system into a cocooning depression.

Chapter 14: **Dream Plain**

He was walking across a mid-western prairie plain. The only man amongst a tribe of women. All of them dressed in buckskin and moccasins.

Moving across the land towards some unknown destination. He was just following when their paths crossed with another tribe of women. So directly did they intersect that he was brushing shoulders with them as they passed. And while Daniel felt the gravitational pull of the group he was traveling with, he stopped when he made eye contact with a young petite brunette at the back of her group. She turned her head, gazing back longingly over her shoulder, but kept walking. Daniel stood still and yearned for her touch.

"Come along Daniel, you can have any one of us." It was the voice of the matriarch telepathically calling in his head.

"But… But I want her…" As he said this the groups were now almost out of sight of one another. Small dots on the horizon. Brief disappointment and longing was erased as they came to a cliff-face overlooking a tropical island. A paradise beach in complete contrast from the dusty earthy plain.

Daniel dived off the cliff and swam through the air as though in water. Flying in full loop de loops. Joyous and ecstatic besides colourful tropical fish, there was nothing more natural than the propulsion of energy from his feet, or inhaling deeply of oxygen rich water.

Landing on the beach there was no one else with him, and all disappointment of not getting the girl had been forgotten.

Chapter 15: One Sentence to Describe the Man

Wisps of his dream were floating and dissipating in his mind as he was awakened by Percival and taken through the routine similar to that of the previous week.

Evacuation of the bowels to seated meditation. Hot water and lemon followed by physical practice. And after the effort and concentration of deep breathing and yoga postures, a cleansing shower.

Daniel walked into the kitchen quiet and calm.

"I've got an answer for the type of man I'd like to become." Percival was at the sink rinsing some fresh mint under the tap.

"Let's hear it."

"You know that feeling when you're in bed and you get to that perfect level of warmth and comfort, and then you remember that you forgot to brush your teeth?"

Percival chuckled a bit "Yeah I know that feeling."

"Well I want to be the type of man that gets up to brush his teeth even though everything is gravitating him not to."

Putting some frozen berries in the blender, Percival stopped mid-movement and turned to Daniel, a look nothing short of admiration shining in his face.

"Now that is a man worth knowing." After a brief instant he went back to placing the berries in the blender and peeling bananas for the shake.

For Daniel, he didn't know what to say after that. Agreeing with him didn't really seem all that appropriate considering he was talking about himself. The statement stood alone as closure. The next first step was now taken and it would not be dwelled upon.

They drank their morning smoothies. Percival making his various "Mmm" sounds at every swallow, and Daniel staring into his purply pink drink with specks of green, wondering what it was next that he needed to do. It sure as hell wasn't to get dressed and go to work.

CHAPTER 16: When in Doubt... Clean.

"The next step is not figuring out where you need to go, or what your purpose is. The next step is simply preparing yourself and the body for that eventuality. Your boat is in dry-dock after some heavy storms and there's a lot of repairs and barnacles to clean off the hull."

"You use a lot of ocean analogies eh Percival?"

"Do they get my point across?"

"You mean do I understand what you're talking about? Yeah I guess I do."

"Good then, that's all that matters to me. If you can gain perspective of where I am coming from, then that is another reference point for you to figure out your own position. If I thought talking in gibberish would somehow be of assistance to you, then you bet your ass I'd be doing my best Jabberwocky impersonation."

"Fair enough... So?"

"So what?"

"So what's the next step?"

"You're asking me?"

"Yeah I guess I am."

"Great. Then the next step is to clean house."

"What, like dusting and vacuuming?"

"It'll be therapeutic beyond measure Daniel. Your life has not necessarily been your own up to this point. You've unwittingly been feeding your energy into a world that does not give you a return on your investment."

"What does that mean?"

"It means that we're going to start building the environment which is more conducive to the man who gets up to brush his teeth when everything is stacked against him. Does a fish that has always swum in a dirty aquarium know that the aquarium has been dirty the whole time?"

"Why are you handing me a scrub brush?"

"To start, you get the bathroom."

"Of course I do. How silly of me."

"Lemon batter, get at 'er"

An hour of nose to the grindstone type work had the bathroom almost sparkling. It also had Daniel needing a break. He walked down to the kitchen to grab a drink.

"Whoa, whoa, whoa! What are you doing with the television?!"

"Get back to cleaning the bathroom."

"You have me scrubbing the bathtub and you're filching my entertainment system?"

"Did you scrub the toilet?" Percival was taking down the 60" plasma screen off the wall that it was mounted on.

"No I didn't, I was coming down for a drink first." Looking around him, wires were neatly rolled up on top of speakers, and where the PS2 used to be was nothing but a space. "Where the fuck is the playstation?"

"Don't forget to get behind the toilet." To Daniel, the room where he would host and be hospitable was now desolate and sad. ...*Everyone that has ever come over loved this place. They loved it!*...

"Yeah gotcha, the back of the toilet, why are you taking the T.V.?"

"When was the last time you were inspired to create something?"

"Like what?"

"Like anything Daniel. Create a short story, draw a picture, play an instrument, even make a nice meal."

"Well I thought about writing my Mum a letter this morning."

"When was that exactly?"

"During the yoga practice."

"In the act of creating your yoga practice you were inspired to create a letter."

"Yeah."

"And when is the last time you watched T.V. and were inspired to make something?" Daniel's jaw dropped open slightly and his eyes rolled back in his head as he thought back.

"That's the exact face you make when watching the T.V. no doubt."

"Alright I get your point."

"ALREADY?!" Percival was clearly surprised.

"Sure. I feel the shut down happen, and to be honest I don't like myself all that much when I've sat in front of the boob tube for a couple hours. It's just a habit I've had since childhood"

"Your ability to let go of shit is uplifting Dude."

"Hey thanks P"

"Now go scrub the shitter. It's buckethead time."

Chapter 17: Faith and Consistency

These were their days for the next weeks. Daniel, feeling invigorated, would jump into these activities. Simple things like preparing a meal, washing the dishes, or walking to the fruiterie. At the other end, finding himself utterly consumed with a morose defeatist attitude, brooding and wretched to the point of destruction. Riding the waves of his positive emotions like some beautiful dolphin at the prow of a ship, to drowning in the fetid filth of his negativity.

In his inspiration he understood completely what he was doing. The body in this state exuded a compulsion to act. Outside of the inspiration was a black cloud. In that dearth he could not even remember at a cellular level what it felt like to feel good or even want good in his life. Overwrought with despair that those wisps of positive memories were nothing but a ruse to fool him. Consumed in the mud bog of ugly thoughts was like having the flu. He just couldn't remember what it was like to be healthy with a clear sinus. And then he'd feel good again.

It was towards the end of summer now. Montreal was still very much alive with festivals and colour, camera carrying tourists and road construction.

Daniel's body had changed. To him it was a slight shift, to someone who would not have seen him in many months, it would have seemed to be a transformation of a shocking extent. Exercise, anatomical study, sleep, and an enormous change in the routine and ingredients of his diet had Daniel feeling more life than ever before. So much so that at times he thought his head would spontaneously combust.

Chapter 17(a): **Welcome to the Grind**

There's a reason the previous chapter is so short, and it's because to you, the reader, there is no entertainment value in reading the same thing over and over again. Fair enough, in the name of brevity and for entertainments sake, we understand that another 100 or thousand or ten thousand chapters of the same thing would not get read. But the reader must understand that while the story of this book is the journey, the real journey for the reader (That's YOU!) is in what is not gone into detail. For it is in the BORING and FUCKING TEDIOUS repetition of these small important things that will actually activate and facilitate lasting and meaningful change in the individual. It's not glamorous, and it sure as shit won't be plastered on any billboards with your face as the poster child. It's hard, thankless, embracing the grind, work. Period.

Chapter 18: Intelligence in Creation

They were sat on the metro going north to Jean Talon Market. The train car was sparsely populated with the rush being in the other direction.

"Did you know the body produces fat to protect itself?"

"Sure, my love handles will keep me afloat when I'm drowning." Daniel was smiling because the comment came from out of left field. Percival had been quiet since they left the house a half an hour before.

At first these silences unsettled Daniel greatly. He would blabber on and on about anything and everything. Nothing was too trivial or obscure. Asking questions about Percival's story, politics, or some random nonsense about something that was happening at that moment. And then one day while Daniel was talking about… he couldn't even remember what it was, Percival wound up and punched him straight in the face. It wasn't a haymaker but it had enough force in it to toggle his brain. Percival had actually made the movements very deliberate so that Daniel saw it coming.

The sound of the knuckles on his face shut him up and brought conversations around them on the café patio they were sitting on, to a halt. There was no movement from anything or anyone for 10 seconds. Even the wind ceased.

"Daniel…" Percival had a calm and kind look on his face "… shut up."

Since then he was a touch more aware of what he was saying and the relevance, if any, that it carried. No need to risk another rat under his left eye.

"Stress is hard on the body. Modern technological western world is full of stress. Right down to the food people are consuming. So John Q Guy or Jane X Girl not only has an exterior stressful job that doesn't inspire them and has to sit in traffic with all the other John Q's and Jane X's who are equally uninspired by their professions, they are also putting their bodies under stress from the inside by eating foods which inflame the body and make it work harder."

"So where does fat production come in?"

"Imagine your body in perfect form. Envision yourself as the Vitruvian Man. Perfect muscular proportion and balance, and let's say that that reflects heath."

"OK." Daniel was seeing his image in a kilt and Braveheart makeup.

"Now what gets one to that form is an interior system rich and efficient, with proper usage and placement of said bodily vessel in its chosen environment. Starting with the exterior environment, if there is a lot of stress, the body will act in a number of ways to buffer itself from that acidity."

Jean Talon Market is a traditional farmer's market. Stall after stall of intentionally placed colours to seduce the senses. Reds and greens and yellows brilliantly contrasted by the mainly generic blacks and greys of the shopper's attire.

The market is alive though, no mistake. It is a place to meet and be met. The Gallic flair of a generous smile and arm gesticulations by the vendors brings a constant buzz. To one more accustomed to the lifeless shopping down aisles of salad dressings and cereals it is quite the experience. This is not just getting food to stock the fridge or pantry, this is meeting the people directly responsible for putting it there.

"Fat is not a bad thing, it is insulation from harm."

"So you're telling me that guy's spare tire is a good thing?"

"Yes Daniel I am. Fat is a solution. Just like your love handles are good for you in a certain way. That insulation from the outside environment protects the entire form like a diver in a full body wetsuit. The skin as our largest organ does a lot of things to protect us, but it needs reinforcement or help from time to time."

"OK I can see that."

"Good. Now the more interesting thing is how the body needs to protect itself from what is ingested, if what is swallowed is either toxic or inflammatory to the system."

"Can you give me an example?"

"I can give you hundreds, but yes I will give you one. Coca-Cola or Pepsi has a ph-level of 3.5, there and about. That is a pretty corrosive acidic level. This goes into the body and the body needs to insulate itself from that. So it appropriates calcium from the bones to make sure it doesn't cause too much damage."

"Doesn't orange juice have a ph-level of about 3.5?"

"It does Daniel, but you're comparing something that grows in nature to something that by all intents and purposes has its home in a laboratory. And not only that, but imagine you did drink a couple liters of orange juice every day for a week or two. What do you think would happen?"

"I'd be pooing pee."

"Burning poo pee Daniel. You'd probably have canker sores in your mouth and red sores on your anus from all the wiping." They were both laughing in the classic frat boy way when dealing with sex or bodily functions. "Orange juice is not bad for you Daniel, hell under the right circumstances Coca-Cola might not be entirely negative, but too much will initiate a counter balancing effect. The toxins that the body can't deal with and can't get rid of are fat-soluble. Which means they dissolve in fat. So the body wraps these toxins in fat and stores them off to the side until such time that it feels like it can get rid of them.

The problem is that some people keep on eating the same toxins so the system stores more off to the side."

"So my love handles are my body's way of dealing with my poor choices?"

"Precisely."

"And when I start making the right choices the body will respond appropriately?"

"It already has Daniel. You feeling sick to your stomach at times is a great thing. It shows the body is getting rid of some of its older stored crap."

"Me feeling like the ass-end of life is a good thing?" His face was half wincing and half nostalgic at the thought of some of his heavy times in the past weeks.

"What, you think the fat you're burning off is full of roses and fairy dust?"

"Touché."

"You just made an interesting comment that I'd like to clarify."

"OK. Touché?"

"Don't be a smart ass. You mentioned poor choices and right choices, which was amazing. Couldn't have labeled them better myself. But when you say right choices we're not talking about the opposite of wrong, we're talking about perfect. The perfect decision Daniel, and the perfect choice in the instant that you're there. They're not always the same day to day."

"What if I don't know what the perfect choice is?"

"We're beginning to ensure that that is almost irrelevant. You have the equation…"

"Plus the minus, minus the plus."

"Right. You have that and certain new ways of protecting or uplifting yourself. The repertoire of tools and wisdom at your disposal is accumulating."

Daniel did feel more… Well he just felt more. More present, more grounded, more "me".

"But let's say you do get into a situation where you are paralyzed."

His mind immediately shot to standing in Dick's office listening to the tirade. He felt the same sick slimy filthy sensation rise up in his belly just below his sternum.

"Any decision Daniel, any decision to act is going to be better than helpless paralysis."

"What if it's not true?! What if the situation is totally crazy?! What if everything I do makes it worse?!" His heart was racing. Feeling the caustic shame of being escorted out of the building.

"Daniel. Daniel! Do you feel that? Can you see how you just dropped into reaction and the victim?"

"I'm feeling really unsettled."

"OK, so get a feel of what this is like for you. Get a perspective on where you are when your energy is like this."

"What do I feel like? I feel like shit and want to get out of it."

"Excellent. And then what?"

"I… I don't know, I guess it feels like I've been labeled or plastered with some sticky film."

"Good, and…"

"And it's not mine! I'm restricted. It feels like it's leeching from me. Making me feel more tired, more fatigued, more… helpless." The realization dawned on him. Feeling helpless is the immediate precursor to giving up. Another small ray of light was piercing his darkness.

"Daniel even right now your body is trying to deal with the stress and strain of the reactionary state you just dropped into. Understand this, if the body were to release what is stored all in one shot, at the very least you would get extremely sick, and at the other end of the spectrum you would be dead."

He hadn't thought of it like that before. It gave him pause.

"So fat seems like a Trojan Horse then?"

Percival's ears perked up at this. "Interesting. Elaborate."

"The body stores the fat outside the gates of Troy. All of the toxins that have ill will remain confined there until they are brought inside the cities walls."

"I like it. Then what?"

"Well out come the Ithatoxins,"

"Clever." Percival responded to Daniel's head inclination.

"And if the person doesn't know about them they run roughshod."

"I'd never thought of the Iliad in that way before."

"But how about this!" He was getting a little more animated and excited in his tone. "If Hector's father, uhhh, what was his name?"

"Priam."

"Yeah, if Priam knew about it all, he could have dealt with the problem with minimal casualties and saved Troy."

"Haha you've just written the alternate ending to one of the original books of western literature."

"Imagine if they would have brought the Trojan Horse into the city and smoked them out."

"Dude, Achilles was in there. Better leave it outside."

"Yeah. Good point."

Chapter 19: French/English, Francais/Anglais

The buzz of French surrounded them with intermittent breaks of English or Spanish, Arabic or Italian.

It was one place where Daniel felt more mature, so to speak, than Percival. Having an adequate grasp of the language, he could speak with the vendors in their mother tongue. After a couple years of studying and courses provided for by his former employer, he knew he had turned a corner in his ability when he made his first joke.

Learning a new language, especially for a uni-lingual Englishman, is terribly humbling. In English Daniel was, at the time, a confident 25 year-old man, in French however he was more like an 8 year-old boy.

As he progressed he was able to appreciate more greatly the role French culture played in buffering everything from the more potent aspects of the North American corporate capitalism. There was definitely the presence of big box stores, but somehow they didn't seem so prominent. Or important. Which meant that in each part of the city there would be that gem of a small family run boulangerie (bakery), café, or restaurant.

At it's best the English/French cohesion (or French/English as some would contest) was efficient without trying to homogenize everything. The spirit of joie de vie meaning people were happy to spend a little more to get their special pastry or a quality loaf of bread.

Percival for his part though, acted the same with people he could and could not necessarily speak with. His demeanor was casual and jovial. As always his quick smile was more disarming than the language barrier was an issue.

Chapter 20: The Making of a Man

"Even not choosing is a choice. Going along with the flow is as much a decision as stepping up. There's a big difference between choosing to stay in stillness letting things unfold, and being paralyzed or impotent to make action. Choosing paralysis or impotence is a heavy choice though."

Daniel enjoyed coming here to the market, but Percival seemed to be on another level. Engaging the vendors in easy conversation, leaving them with bigger smiles than when they had arrived, and taking away another basket of berries or bunch of carrots.

They were laden down with bags overflowing. Leafy greens and vegetables, baguettes and raw cheeses, fruits, flowers (Percival said they absorb negative energy), and artisan dark chocolates.

Daniel's diet may have been restricted in terms of processed foods, but they were having such memorable meals.

"This is like sex to me." He was completely serious as he looked at Daniel. "There is so much life here. It's an orgy of the senses. And I'm not just talking about the colourful displays or the constant din of the crowd. Feel it Daniel, feel the entire scenario like a woman in heat wanting to be fucked."

Daniel looked around and saw an old woman with a miniature poodle and a little child throwing a pizza crust and paper plate onto the ground.

"I'm seeing a lot, but very little of it is sexy."

"Sex is more than dick in cunt Daniel."

"Haha you're getting a bit vulgar aren't you?" He was laughing, but in his belly was a warmth of discomfort touched on by the outspoken topic.

"Intentionally blunt in this regard, yes. I'm speaking of the deep celebration of intimate love."

"Not dick in cunt?"

"This whole thing is dick in cunt Daniel. Only it's the phallus of consciousness that penetrates for pleasure. Dancing, undulating, life-sized poetry. Some may see it as a video game, or literature, or sport, or even a movie. I like to think of it as one giant love-fest.

The feminine energy loves to be seen in appreciation. Consciousness being masculine provides the mirror for that beauty.

In the grand scale everything in this physical reality is feminine. Your body included. The watching of this, the aware observer of such beauty is a masculine quality."

"The painting is feminine, the appreciation of the painting is masculine."

"Yes. Great. Now in modern world terms, beauty has become a commodity."

"Hasn't it always been?"

"Yes, but consciousness is also a commodity. Only society doesn't know how to quantify it."

"Which means?"

"Which means that because the populace is largely unaware or uneducated of consciousness as a resource to cultivate inside themselves, they unconsciously seek it out in exterior situations."

"Exterior situations?"

"The general equation for compliments is that if a man gives a compliment to a woman, generally the woman will take the compliment and put it in her pocket like spare change. But if a woman gives a compliment to a man, the initial thought is that he might be able to get a piece of ass."

"Which might be why women so seldom give compliments to strangers."

"Exactly, who wants to give someone a quarter if they keep trying to take your wallet afterwards?"

"Haha, point taken."

"It's a closed circuit. Each person is endowed with masculine and feminine qualities. Beauty and consciousness.

John Q. Guy, emotionally immature and undisciplined, getting recognized by what he perceives to be a beautiful woman is a double whammy. First there's her loveliness, but then there's her consciousness which has seen his traits.

For a guy unschooled in the refinements of the spirit, any response is more than likely laced with desperation."

"The foul cologne."

"The foulest."

"So why do you think that most guys are not… uhm…"

"Men?"

"Haha yeah I guess."

"Well what makes up a man?"

"That's what I thought I was asking you about."

"Don Quixote talks of three levels of mastery in order to create a gentleman. Physically he is healthy and robust. Intellectually he is well lettered and thirsty for knowledge. And finally, and maybe most importantly, he is emotionally secure and self-sufficient."

"That last one is a tough one."

"Damn right it is. And for guys especially there are few, if any, acceptable mainstream outlets to understand their emotional self in a safe and vulnerable way."

"Just hearing the word vulnerable sucks my testicles a little closer to my body." Daniel was trying to be funny.

"Physical prowess? Easy. Intellectual sharpening? Groups are accessible. But something for the emotional quotient?

Right now you have two generally accepted ways to become a man. One is the army and one is sport. The first one doesn't want a man, it wants an automaton that follows orders and stays between the lines. The second is not that much better after a certain point. In both instances it is a rarity for these men to sit down earnestly and honestly to discuss, probe, or otherwise share their emotions."

"So where do we go?"

"Daniel, finding emotional stability is not a place or a group. Growing one's balls is being present and honest with those things that make us most uncomfortable."

"I feel like I've been doing a good job of that lately."

Percival stopped in his tracks. Daniel walked a few steps ahead before it registered. As he stopped and turned, Percival's bags were on the pavement, and had walked over to wrap him in a hug.

Not a big bear hug that a dad would give, overly squeezing to cover up the insecurity and desperate need for the expression of such emotion.

Not a dude hug with the three hard pats on the back and then the release, to cover up the insecurity and desperate need for the expression of such emotion.

This was a hug that was firm and constant, but gentle and tender. A hand at his middle back pressed deeply and brought their sternums together. It was, to put it simply, intimate.

Two men standing in an embrace, one with arms at his sides holding bags of groceries in each hand. The other, leaning into, but also seemingly holding up, the other.

At first Daniel sort of laughed at the hug he was receiving. *Percival being Percival*, he thought. As it continued however his mind and discomfort amplified.

…What is he doing? Everybody's watching. This is really weird…

Seconds kept ticking into a minute, or was it two?

"I love you Daniel." It was said delicately. The sound of his voice could also be felt by Daniel as a vibration passing in his chest.

That tipped him over the edge. As much as it was the words, it was the deep resonant feeling that Percival actually MEANT those words.

… Totally weird! What does he think I'm gay? I know he doesn't. Does he? I'm not gay. Not that there's anything wrong with that but I'm not!…

His balls really were now in full retreat into his abdomen.

"Whoa whoa whoa…" Daniel pulled straight back with wide eyes and ashen face. "Uhh… I don't think that… what I mean to say is that, uhh… you might have gotten the wrong impression with what I, uhm"

"So you think you've been doing a good job of being present and honest with those things that make you most uncomfortable?" The question brought traction to his spinning tires. Percival's entire demeanor had changed to a more masculine standoffish nature.

"Wait, what?"

"You've still got a long way to go Sonny boy, you can only accept as much love as you give to yourself. This goes for anyone."

"I can only let someone love me as much as I love myself."

"And vice versa. How can you ever love another with a gallon of love when your vessel is only capable of holding a thimble full?"

"I don't know about that, I feel like I've loved some women pretty deeply."

"Bullshit. You hemorrhaging dependence was a projection of your emotional desperation."

"Fuck you!" he was hurt as he thought about Jenny. About Katherine. And Stephanie. Those MEANT something.

"Would you have died for those loves?"

"Of course I would have." An unconscious pumping up of his chest happened.

"And what would that have been worth? Handing over a limp dick impotent masculinity to the Alter of Woman. Who the fuck would want that?"

"No, but…"

"The carcass of some shitty lover that those women would have to carry around with them."

"Yeah, but…"

"Which is a major factor as to why these relationships failed in the first place. These women could trust in their own masculine energy more than they could trust in your own childish man-boy."

"OK, I get it, but…" He had his hands up, palms facing out in the form of a traffic cop giving the all-stop.

"Dying for someone is not an expression of love Daniel, LIVING IS!" He screamed the last two words. Loud enough for people in passing to turn and look in their direction. And as they looked, Percival looked back at them "Hello. Bonjour." Which evoked little responses of small smiles. "The real gift to your loves is to forge and purify yourself into the absolute quintessential gentleman. Now THAT is a gift."

"Emotionally secure and self-sufficient…" Daniel stated this as though reciting a couple ingredients for a recipe he intended to prepare.

"More and more you're well versed in how to take care of yourself physically. That's easy, scientific even. Intellectually, is a matter of study and mastering the object of study.

The real work is just beginning. You asked me before where one goes to secure his emotional welfare? Well he goes into the deepest, darkest, and most unknown areas of his life. In short, he goes in."

…*Oh shit…*

"Oh shit."

"Exactly. If you don't like farting in the company of others, women especially, this little inward journey you're about to take is going to be uncomfortable, humid and stinky. It requires an openness and honesty about your shit. Because you're not only dealing with the emotional immaturity of subjects like fighting, sex and bowel movements, you're having to assimilate them at an intellectual level as well."

"What do you mean?"

"It means stepping into the fear of being made fun of, being put down by the masculine, and the very real fear of being abandoned and rejected by the feminine." Daniel winced at the word 'abandoned'. "If it's been repressed for a while, it will have de-evolved from its initial stage. Which means a wild, hairy, vengeance seeking energy."

"OK, so what do we do?" More and more he trusted the line and direction Percival was taking. Before he might have done what he was told, but begrudgingly. Now there was a willingness to see the unknown outcome of whatever scenario was laid before him.

"Have you ever had to pull a hairball out of your shower drain?"

"Yeah, it's grey and filmy and disgusting."

"Feels pretty good to pull it out though eh?"

"Well... yeah, I guess it does."

"And the water flows more freely down the drain afterwards."

"True."

"So we're going to clean up your drains."

"Like janitors of the universe." Daniel, standing erect like a superhero, had a big grin on his face as he said this. They laughed for the rest of the walk home envisioning the various powers of Janitorman.

Chapter 21: **Self-Activation**

One has to be in a certain mood to read or write poetry. The symbolism can come across as flighty and self-serving to one who is not in the heart-song.

For Daniel, writing had been an expressive form visited in high school or during a romantic tryst. He loved it, even romanticizing that part of himself in adulthood. It was a vulnerable place though. Beyond just saying "I'm happy" or "I'm sad", poetry demands a state of introspection deeper than the intellect. So it was seldom he would visit his muse.

It was the cleansing tool Percival would have him use in the coming weeks. And at first it was agony. An ominous wall, bearing down and intimidating his fledgling steps. Half an hour of sitting in front of a blank page would bring 95% berating judgment for each snippet of flow. Swimming in a stream of self-directed venom for his inability and inaction.

… Hadn't it been easier before all this? …

As tough and tactically precise as Percival was in the morning practice and regimen, he was equally soft and soothing in his requests to "Open your heart Daniel, this is good, accidents and missteps can lead you to your love."

And then… it came. In one long streaming otherworldly rush. Word after word, Rhyme upon vision, vision into metaphor, metaphor into heart song. A dirty heart song.

> *Hey! Smell that?*
> *Smells like consumerism.*
> *Biff baff baby boomerism.*

Mmm...smells great.

Makes me want to procreate.

Salivate. Quarter pounder with cheese I don't need the plate.

I'll just throw out the wrapper.

Nature's my crapper.

Women's got power I fear so I slap her.

<<SMACK>> Bitch.

Hey! Hear that?

Sounds like a modern prophesy.

Doesn't matter too much that it's based on hypocrisy.

Patriarchal warrior, dominating control.

Put your mothers on alert, and your sons on patrol.

A generation of children raised in a mans body.

Third rock planet Earth is my porta-pottie.

Objectify females and squeeze that hot tottie.

Slut.

Mmm feel that?

Solid steel metallic.

Let everyone know my anger is phallic.

Oh yeah baby. Rock hard!!

I'm the big man so I'll stand on guard.

En guarde!!!

You make me uncomfortable so I call you a retard.

In my mind's eye you can either bar-b-que it or broil it.

Everyone's having a good time at the party so I spoil it.

The backyard's my toilet.

My ideal lady should be trustworthy, obedient
and loyal SIT!

Tramp.

Hey! See this?

It's my legacy.

Unabashed, unbiased depravity.

What do you think?

I'm doing my best to get us just past the brink.

What did you bring?

Nothing? Oh, I don't count love and peace and all
those hippie things.

That's just worthless trash.

I'm more interested in cold hard cash.

Mortgage my future as I rape, cut and slash.

Notching my bedpost with all the sex that I've
snatched.

Whore.

What? What's everyone looking at me like that for?

You're the ones who let me trample the backs of
the downtrodden and poor.

Ummm...I'm feeling a little uncomfortable...
soooo... let's... go... to... war!

Hey! See this?

It's the wrong direction.

Filling my pockets with a disappearing collection.

A new zoo to display my weakness as power.

Tick tocking it down to the final witching hour.

BONG BONG BONG!!!

It's patriotism.

I'm a big fan of human creationism.

God put us here.

Spread a message of either hatred or fear.

Call anyone different either "Hitler" or "Queer".

It's not just fiction.

I have an inbred right to duty dereliction.

I ain't got no need for using proper diction.

Why? Because I'm just a boy in a mans body.

Won't admit my mistakes, just praise Goddy.

PRAISE JEEEESUS!!!!

Jesus. Our worlds falling to pieces.

Let my unnecessary accessories fall through the cracks and the creases.

Play catch with my nephews, and secrets with my nieces.

Cunt.

But hey! Smell that again?

Smells like consumerism.

Biff baff baby boomerism.

Mmm... smells great.

Makes me want to procreate.

Dominate. Pumping oil and gas we need another interstate.

Let's make history poverty.

Forget past lessons and big brother our liberty.

Because I am the modern man.

Quarterly reports. Five year plans. Modern man.

5 minute managers. Media bans. Modern man.

Healthy orange hue from my fake and bake tan. Modern man.

My birth worth more on earth than what the universe spans. Modern man.

Temper incontinence with diuretics and bran.
Modern man.

Temper incompetence with, "Don't blame me.
I'M *just following orders" and then hold up*
your hands. Modern man.

There is no Renaissance, just the Bible and
C-span. Modern man.

Everything's alright cause I am the Modern man.
Everything's hunky cause I am the Modern man.
Everything's dorry cause I'm the Modern man.
There's no need to say sorry
Put your faith in my hands cause I'm the
Modern man.

Better yet, put your tithe in my hands cause I'm
the Modern man.

Modern man.
Modern man.
Modern man.

Percival read through the words once, and then twice. Putting the pages to the right of Daniel he said.

"That's great Daniel, really great... but... we already know all that."

Daniel's shoulders dropped. Not because he was crushed, but because he knew he was right. This was a stream without solutions. It was a finger pointing at the muck saying "Look, this is dirty!" But the seal had been broken. The subtle critique was an injection to do more. To be more! A la Dead Poet's Society.

This was his arms wide. No holding back. He sat up, grabbed his pen and was about to start writing again.

"Not yet bud. Let's go. We have to get rolling."

"Yeah but I'm feeling really inspired. I want to ride this out."

"I know you are. Remember this feeling next time you come to sit down. For now we're going to run on this inspiration."

So they did. Running through Parc Lafontaine. Around the water with its pigeons and gulls and fowl, passing couples laying in the shade in dozing love embraces, they ran. The iron electric taste in his lungs, lactic acid fatigue in his muscles, heavy feet getting heavier. And amidst the crush and flush of more strides came what had been lacking in years of meeting resistance. Yes. Yes had come. Yes to the ache, yes to the experience, yes to resistance itself that, for his whole adult life he had been avoiding.

No. The symbol of the victim. No. The interior statement of one who denies what is happening in the misdirected hope that it might alter what it is. No. Which places another barrier between lover and beloved.

So he said yes and felt grief and apology at being away from his heart for so long. Interwoven with his 'Yes', was "I'm sorry". Acknowledging the folly that kept him so distant from his heart.

The forgiveness was immediate. The heart holds no malice, it simply wants us back. Infinitely patient it awaits us to simply stop and listen.

Daniel was in the clouds. Calm and quiet in the pulse and pump of perpetuating gait with his brother.

… *Thank you…*

He only knew he was saying thank you to everything. To anything. Finding rebirth into life through his own trajectory, and the more he said thank you, said yes, some other source would spring forth in aid. Presenting itself in forms of memories internally, or synchronous smiles or movements from his external surroundings.

He allowed the light of Percival's profession of love to actually shine into his shineshine thing. And where before there was shame or insecurity, he found grace.

Stopping at a bench near a water fountain Daniel was transfixed by a little dark haired girl, no older than a year and a half. She was walking. That's it, just walking. It was a new experience for her, and the absolute joy on her face at being able to do something which he found to be so simple, imprinted upon him. The gift of locomotion and the next step. The father close, but not too close behind, in a happy world of his own listening to her squeals of delight.

"I felt a wall bearing over me when I was writing." Their deep gasping breaths were slowing down.

"OK, and then what?"

"Well, I think it might have been a wall of old stories that I had built up as protection, but that protection was also cutting me off from new experiences." His forehead was creased in the perplexity of a new puzzle. "The poem came forth when I deconstructed the barrier. The wall became fuel."

"I like that analogy."

"Yeah the wall isn't bad. It's just grown out of its service in a certain way. Like a grotesque monument to a bygone era."

"So now the question is what has that wall been protecting you from?"

"He looked skyward. The answer had come immediately but he was still tentative to voice it so quickly.

"… As near as I can make it… I think… I think it's been protecting me from the vulnerability of my love." It took his breath away to verbalize it.

"Bingo."

His mind started unraveling at an incredible speed. The density of emotions were unfolding in a path. Story after self-professed story. Sitting at the centre of his spider web, people, events and symbols dangling like dewdrops and jewels on the strands. A vision of his entire world, his entire life, was a self-fulfilling prophesy. He had attracted and created this menagerie. All as a curriculum of learning. He was the author, protagonist, antagonist and story. A low-grade Rumi poem.

It was a new phase of locomotion to discover. The more he stepped down the path, the more it laid itself at his feet.

Daniel suddenly felt very tired. Comprehending at long last, just how long he had been on energetic rations for love and contentment. It was a lamenting wave. The sickly sweet mourning process.

They walked the rest of the way back home. Daniel's nervous system replete with weariness made a beeline for his bed and sunk into a deep sleep. It was the surest thing he knew to do.

Chapter 22: The New Normal

As like every other morning, groggy eyed, Daniel awoke to Percival's bright visage.

"How do you do it man? How are you this energized and happy at 6 in the morning?"

"I've made the routine that we're going through the norm. My nervous system is not only clean, its roots at the very tips are extracting energy and assimilating it in divine order."

"Yeah but you're ALWAYS good."

"Little tip for you, I'm not good or great or exceptional, I'm normal."

"So what does that do for you?"

"There's fitness fanatics who work out diligently, religiously even, for 6 days a week, controlling their food intake, counting calories, taking supplements, and making superhuman efforts… and on the 7th day God created the "Cheat Day.""

"Haha, I've known a few of those guys."

"Being REALLY good means at some point you're going to be REALLY bad."

"And that's not good."

"Haha, it is what it is. There's a lot to learn in the extremes, but there is also a lot of hardships and aging. It's fun going 100km/hr and then slamming on the brakes, but it puts a major strain on a lot of the cars systems."

"Bald tires."

"Burning oil."

"Leaky transmission."

"Overheated radiator."

"Misaligned wheels."

"I've said it before. We're supposed to feel good ALL THE TIME. That's normal. And if not, then something is wrong and needs to be fixed or attended to."

"That's a tall order."

"Our body is a powerful machine. 100 trillion cells all working together for the betterment of the whole, even if that means dying off. And if parts of us don't want to die, if parts of us don't let go?"

"Well cells that don't die in the body are cancer cells."

"Exactly. Feeling horrible is a signpost to where a cycle has run its course but has stagnated in its completion."

"You've been guiding me in that haven't you?"

"Daniel these immense comatose sleeps you've been having are the nervous system's way to intelligently heal itself. These weeping crying releases are hungry ghosts and vestiges of an old self being laid to rest."

"My grief and mourning is necessary then."

"And valid. We honour those parts of us that have been loyal. This is what allows them to be free." He stopped for a moment and put his hand on Daniel's shoulder. "Daniel, I die all the time. I bury pieces of myself, but I celebrate the fact that I had the honour to know them in the first place."

"And this opens space for you to feel healthy and full of vigour?"

"That's the gift that death gives to life. In the course of human history, each generation has done its best to leave the Earth better than what they found it."

"Standing on the shoulders of giants right?"

"Yeah man, Newton was a wise man. Millions of skin cells die daily so that the next generation can have their time in the sun. The body is the same reflection as the greatest or worst parts of your own human history."

"The microcosm in the macrocosm."

"Yessir, the microcosm in the macrocosm." Daniel loved these pauses in conversation. As though they had come to an end of a verbal chapter. "I think you're ready my friend."

"Ready for what?" Said with no small amount of apprehension. Percival's eyes shone as a spontaneous one syllable laugh left his throat.

Chapter 23: **Mirror Work**

"Straight ahead. Minimize your blinking. Watch yourself." It was just after 4 in the morning. When Daniel protested about getting out of bed. In fact his exact words were "Are you fucking insane?" Percival, like an old fisherman arousing images of his favourite fishing hole simply said that the energy was more clear at this time of day.

"Are you serious?" This was as genuine a question as he had ever asked. "You want me to stand and stare at myself in the mirror?" At least now, Daniel felt, he had definitive proof as to Percival's deteriorating mental state.

"Straight ahead. Minimize your blinking. And watch your self." The last three words were said distinctly separate as he walked out of the room to leave him alone.

The first thing he noticed was just how quiet everything was around him. "Honest" was the word that popped into his head. All the lights were off, but there was a silver essence illuminating the livingroom.

… Is it a full moon?…

The mirror in front of which he stood was full length, leaning slightly against the wall, and had a 6" dark wood square frame. The silhouette of his form was slightly unfamiliar.

… Another trick of the light…

His face was angled and sharper in the half exposed to the window, while the side cast in shadow seemed to deepen and disappear. He was wearing a light blue long sleeve and a pair of basketball shorts. Bare feet hip width apart molded to the floor with palms facing forward in anatomical position.

The conversation began. First in his head, that was normal, he was always talking to himself. Wasn't he? Even with one side of his face in shadow, both eyes were staring back, glistening. Knowing.

… Am I talking with myself? Is that reflection me?…

A very slight forward and back motion started in the soles of his feet as he perceived the balancing up through his legs into the pelvis and low back. His breath lengthened.

… My eyes, that's my face, but it's not my face. Who is that? Who's there?…

A voice popped up from behind the normal flow of thoughts "It's me!" This voice was younger, higher pitch than what he was accustomed to hearing.

He jerked at the outside intrusion. The face staring back at him changed. It was smiling, ever so slightly, his eyes locked gazes with the reflection, as the face looking back grew luminous. He could feel tingling in his fingers. The slight swaying seemed almost out of sync with the movement in the mirror. The smile turned from gentle to mischievous to malevolent in an instant. Another voice came from the back of his head "You piece of shit." He stiffened, a hot flush flared in his chest and skull. It was a predator energy dark and sinister.

… That's not me…

Fear crawled up his back as the air around him got thicker and seemed to menacingly encroach upon him. All his senses went into high alert. Breath was shallow, heartbeat pounding. His face changed to a mask of death. A decrepit old man, sad and war torn, looking to inflict pain.

… If the voice in my head is me, then who's listening?…

Rationally he was trying to assure himself that he was safe.

… I'm just standing in front of my mirror…

A rising venomous sarcastic laughter "Oh no, I wouldn't hurt you." He felt a childishness bullied and frightened. Other voices along with these were in continual cascade. A white noise bustle of the spectrum of his emotions. Most of them, if not all of them, outside the normal range of his comfort zone.

Behind his reactions, behind the temptation to turn tail and run *…Where could I run? It's myself…* Was a more stolid stable nature. A piece of him tired of running. Whether he was fully conscious of it or not, all of his training had forged and committed him to this very moment. He stood his ground and heard an old National Film Board of Canada cartoon from his childhood. The woman's voice quite British and matronly, "Persuasion is better than force."

"You fucking piece of shit"

… Yes …

Another shade of hatred "I'll kill you, you cowardly motherfucker."

… I'm sorry …

It was a whirling maelstrom. Standing in the midst of this anger tornado were his eyes unwavering and witnessing. No avoidance. No scrambling. No cowering. No paralysis. Just watching the insanity unfold like he had watched the path of his story unfold at the end of his run in Parc Lafontaine.

"Worthless no good sack of shit."

… I understand …

And he did. In avoiding abandonment by being the instigator of dismantling a relationship, he had in fact been abandoning his own internal love impulse. This was the tar-like entrails of what Robert Bly termed 'The long black bag we drag behind us.' Daniel, acknowledging and allowing these energies to have their time in the light of his consciousness, was creating a ceremony in healing. He was accepting and welcoming back parts of his self, which had been ostracized and subjected for years.

He began to deepen his breath. At the top of a full inhale he would retain the breath and bring his focus into the grounding of his feet. As though steeling his self for contact with an oncoming wave. The blood pressure in his chest, neck, and head increased until he could not hold it any longer. The release brought on a blood rush and disorientation. A hot flushing went over his body. A respite from the poisoned invective. The rising of the breath again, brought him to a place akin to stasis. Heart pounding in his throat and skull. Holding at the bottleneck of pressure until letting go and sending out the heavier thicker exhale.

It was a shit storm. The harsh judgments of his own ignorance made it that there was no clean way to deal with it.

"The janitors of the universe!" he heard Percival's voice laughing.

"You think you're so cool, no one likes you, you're not worth anything, you have no talent"

… *I forgive you* … The definition of forgiveness being 'Thank you FOR GIVING me this experience'. Forgiveness being a healing of any hurt that one may find to have incurred at the hands of themselves or others. Forgiveness is a healing of one's own bridge to the heart.

"Like I care you inauthentic cunt."

... I love you ... Holding his breath again he could see that all this was just another layer of his self. There were deeper more still water's speaking or getting through. Like a far distant church bell ringing its truth, Daniel understood the salve of its words and began to repeat the mantra being presented to him "The war is over."

... The war is over ...

At first repeating it mentally, he started to whisper the phrase and then grew subtly into the full sound of his normal voice. It surprised him and made him feel a touch silly to hear his voice talk to itself.

'The war is over' meant that, internally, there were no more enemies to his person. Each area of his psyche was valid, loved and welcome. No matter how vicious or ugly they might appear. Some of those pieces would still need to be housebroken, but they had their home now. The days of passive aggressive posturing, or withholding love as weapon, had in this moment been ceased.

He began to let his breath run its own course. The worst of the emotions had abated. There would be more to deal with, but for now he had done all that he could do. Making what surfaced feel safe in its expression. There was the sensation of a dazed calm akin to a young child after an intense tantrum. He turned away from the mirror and walked towards the kitchen where he knew Percival would be. Glancing at the clock on the oven he was a little surprised to see that close to 40 minutes had passed.

Looking up from his book he was reading, Percival walked to the kettle on the stove and started to pour steaming water into a mug. He came back to place the hot water, lemon, ginger and honey before him.

Running a hand through his hair, Daniel took a huge sigh breath.

… Where to begin? …

"The war is over."

"Amen."

It was so nice, Daniel thought, to say something quite random but loaded with symbolism and not have a barrage of questions thrown at him upon the utterance of it. Seconds passed. Percival took a sip of his brew and let out a soft sigh after swallowing.

"There's really no end to it is there?" Daniel more stated this as fact even though it came out in question form.

"Not that I know of."

"In a way I'm always going to need to clean my clothes, or have a shower, or take another breath" He took a pregnant pause "and after I get clean I'm going to get dirty again. In perpetuity."

"Mmhmm." It was a pensive agreement.

"And if there's one thing I realized in watching myself it's that I'm going to have to steward all these parts of myself over and over again."

"Yup. A lot of work."

"It's mine though isn't it? This is what you meant the first day when you said that the Self shall uphold itself by the Self."

"Nicely done." Said in the way of one admiring a good golf shot.

"So if that's the case, then…"

"Yes?" There was that mischievous glint in his eye.

"… Then what's the point?!"

"You mean why are we doing the work?"

"Yeah, I guess."

"You really don't know?"

"No, I honestly have no idea why I should be doing all of this in the first place."

"Which is a very good reason to be doing it."

"C'mon, you know what I mean."

"If you're thinking that by doing all this work Daniel, by putting all of this energy and effort and expenditure forth, that you're supposed to GET something, That you DESERVE something in return, then that's why you're finding yourself so bent out of shape."

"What does that mean?"

"The work IS your gift." He leaned forward. "You've already won the lottery of life. You have a body, you won. You have been given this beautiful vessel with which to experience and celebrate and manifest your gifts." As he was saying this, his hands were oscillating and rotating like a children's magician. "It is an absolute magical time to be alive right now. We could pick up and be in Australia in under 24 hours."

"Yeah." Gazing into his empty mug, his response was tinged with a wistful want to be transported to some beach with bikini-clad blondes.

"When they say that 'It's the journey, not the destination', what they're saying is that the work is your gift, not the reward of someone acknowledging or applauding you. Your reward is that you get to do your life work. That you get to make your world a better place than what you found it yesterday or this morning. Even if it is scrubbing a toilet or folding laundry. To build up a monument in reverence to some divine calling within you to these grand archetypes of LOVE, or LIFE or GOD. This is your gift. That you get to do anything at all. In the words of Kahlil Gibran "Your work is love made visible."

"You're right."

"And you're sitting there telling me you want more? New-age Oliver Twist anyone?"

"No that's not what I meant."

"But it's exactly the attitude you've put out there. The privileged spoiled brat."

"Hey c'mon, be fair, you know I've been doing a lot of work."

"And you want praise for it?"

"No!... Well, maybe. At least a bit of acknowledgment."

"Can't expect to climb to the top of a mountain and have everyone applaud you."

"Is that what I've been doing?"

"Do you believe you have a soul Daniel?"

The question caught him completely off guard.

… Who asks that?…

"Uh… yeah I guess so." His eyebrows furrowed in the response.

"Ok good. This soul would be the pure essence of what you are expressing and creating in this physical realm then correct?"

"You mean is it my higher self? Yeah I'd say so." He was beginning to see where this was going.

"In that description there would need to be a passageway or portal for one to cross into the other."

"OK."

"Now if you're expecting Divine Love of your Soul to appear to you unsoiled as it crosses the threshold of your very human nervous system and body…"

"It's gotta be clean."

"The temple of heaven is within Daniel."

"My expectations are too high."

"You've already gotten everything you require to learn what you need to learn. Whatever you feel not to have received is a pointer to where your work and efforts are best directed."

"The work is my gift." The external affirmation brought about an unconscious nodding of his whole body.

"So let's get to work old man."

It would be wonderful to say that Daniel had an epiphany following his mirror work. Yeah it would have been wonderful to say that.

As it came about, the foreboding threats of disaster were overwhelming.

… You're going to lose it all…

Percival could sense it. His guidance of the postures, nitpicking the slightest alignment cues, was relentless.

"This is it Daniel. Stand your ground here and now, or get lost again."

His body was searing, ears burning.

… Who's talking about me?…

Backbend after backbend. Shoulders straining with an electric compromise. The ordeal physically was compounded by the same internal voices, saying the same things, pressing the same buttons, that had the same effect of impinging and limiting his desire to go beyond their pronouncements. Fear directives. A rhetoric bilge of shame and sin.

To Daniel, he was working as hard as he could. To Percival, Daniel's internal dialogue (He could see it in the creases and expression of his face.) was restricting full and honest effort. Instead of trusting fully to do what instruction was stated, any guidance was going through the filter of his conscious (and convoluted) mind.

"Level up you Fuck!" A precisely placed flagrant swear can be a powerful and beautiful thing. For some reason it made him smile. The honesty of the statement cut right through the insanity of his back and forth into the heart of his driving function. His chest lifted through the ceiling of resistance and a full muscular exhalation cleaned out his abdomen.

Laying down from the backbend he had lost count of how many he had done.

"Good. Again."

Slight hesitation, slight reticence to go back in.

"That's not a question Daniel!" Boom, up he went. Shoulders restricting in a different place, legs shaking at a different speed, and an ever increasing need to laugh.

Where was he? It wasn't Montreal. It wasn't 2013. It wasn't even on his radar to think about it. This is here and now. Without time, without space. No acting, no fakeness, no masks. As true a reflection of what comprised his metal as there is.

"Good. Again." So he did. Grounding the hands and feet. Malleable rooting through his mat. He pressed to the crown of his head, readjusted, and then drove up into his ceiling again.

… The Sistine Chapel must be amazing…

A creative space beyond male and female. Without creed or colour or age. An ancient legacy of humanity was the source. No thoughts. Just a feeling of being connected to a giant inclusive movie.

The laughter came immediately. Whatever it was, it was extremely comical. Or perhaps better stated, it was extremely not serious. None of it. All of it. The physicality of repeating backbends, the emotional turmoil and situation of losing his job, this random relationship with a man that had taken up the lion's share of his time, effort and energy in recent months.

From some quiet windless place inside of him, massive waves of laughter rolled out. A golden monk in robes and sandals bellowing fits of jolly tears.

… *This is a charade. What a wonderful and intricate play to be cast in…*

Seeing beyond the veil of his ignorance was divine order. People that had "Done me wrong." Had only been playing their part in the grand play. Every shred of memory had been integral in his return to this point, and the space that he had found himself in, this space coming from before his creation, seemed to be saying "Did you have a good time?"

The lunacy of his judgmental self, like an ingrown hair doing the opposite of what its intention was, dropped its need for control.

This is where it's wonderful to write that Daniel had his epiphany. A ridiculous gut-busting awakening to the illusion of separateness. Fear had kept him holed up in mental masturbations. Now, NOW, in this feeling of a loving source, the thought of "Losing it all" was amusing beyond belief. It was all his anyway. The quest to fill his emotional void with physical possessions was fruitless at a fundamental level.

… No wonder having more made me feel less. Made me feel less in control…

Wearing fear in the form of a wristwatch and anxiety as a t-shirt printed with the phrase "Abandonment issues". ("Now that is an honest t-shirt! We'll make millions. Get your inner truth dysfunctional child t-shirt now! Only 29.95$ Mine would say 'Please love me." Percival would say later upon hearing the recount.)

His laughter would begin to ebb, softly waning, before catching another perspective of his farcical actions. Which would unload another round of hysterical giggles. Memories of laughing like this in childhood were so present. The incoherent gibberish of trying to relate what was so funny cramped the already aching stomach muscles that had been racked in uncontrollable spasms and contractions for minutes.

CHAPTER 24: I Choose...

It was with the leftovers of the practice that Daniel went to sit down and write. That's all he wanted to do.

"You don't want breakfast?"

"I'm full to overflowing right now P."

"You sure?"

"Yeah, I can feed myself in more ways than just food. I'm hungry to write."

Percival took a deep and appreciative inhale.

"Thanks man."

"For what?" Daniel was uncertain why he was being thanked.

"Just for choosing to do your work."

"Oh... yeah, no problem."

9am and Daniel had already been up for 5 hours, all of them at the highest amount of clarity and efficiency he could remember.

... This must be what it is to be running clean...

Sitting at his desk and the writing flowed, as it had before, but this time there was a softer touch to his words. Even if at first the words were laced with curses, it was a wise and knowing proclamation. Coming from a place of experience from the end of the poem rather than the beginning.

> *Yeah I've told God to fuck off.*
> *My spirit bit it hard, and then it slowly sucked*
>   *it soft.*

I couldn't grasp the gifts he was handing.
I wouldn't comprehend the faith she was demanding.
They didn't understand that it was all just a big misunderstanding.

So I fell from grace.
Floated in the abyss of void, and the void of unspace.

I entered my loneliness.
If the burden I bore were only less.
Only less.
If only my loneliness were only less.

I gave the Almighty the big "fuck off".
So my spirit bit it hard, and then it slowly sucked it soft.

I brought Jesus to task for my aching.
I thought Allah's words to be fraudulent and faking.
They didn't partake in the mistake I was mistaking.

So I fell from grace.
Floated in the abyss of void and the void of unspace.

I entered my impotence.
There was no sense of consequence.
No sense.
My sense of consequence was nonsense.

I told them all to go fuck off.
So my spirit bit it hard and then it slowly sucked
*   it soft.*

I said I'd be my very own savior.
To behave how I like, and like my behavior.
They weren't too crazy about my craziness getting
*   crazier.*

So I fell from grace.
Floated in the abyss of void and the void of
*   unspace.*

I lost my compassion.
There was no flash in my passion.
No flash.
My flash of compassion had ceased to be flashing.

So I kept on saying, "fuck off".
And my spirit bit it hard and then it slowly sucked
*   it soft.*

I went on sabbatical.
My path was errant, erratic and fanatical.
The bad that I bade had become badly radical

And I fell from grace.
Floating in the abyss of void and the void of
*   unspace.*

I entered in melancholic.
A stage of rage in my personal plague bubonic.
Catatonic
The Daniel I was drowning was a negative spirits
  alcoholic.

But never once did they acknowledge my
  embittered fuck off.
Because their knowledge kept them solid and their
  love light kept them soft.

They waited with patience and poise and wisdom.
There was no offense noted in the fact that I
  dissed 'em.
Forgiveness was given before I knew of the
  forgivening.

So I let in what I missed.
Felt them in the midst of my heart and the heart
  of their midst.

I entered my devotion.
My desolate desert was now my emotional ocean.
Their ocean.
My emotional devotion was a dose in their ocean.

They waited for my tantrum to permanently
  shove off.
Then their knowledge kept me solid and their love
  light ever soft.

I was presented with victuals.
Started to learn the blessing of private prayer
rituals.
They hadn't inhabited my individual habituals.

So I let in what I missed.
Felt them in the midst of my heart and the heart
of their midst.

I entered my salvation.
The medication of my station was in the
meditation.
Meditating.
My salvation in creation was in silent meditation.

They viewed my indiscretions from a perch way
up, aloft.
Then their knowledge kept them solid and their
love light ever soft.

Never once had they stopped with their offering.
Never once did they suffer the slight of that 'fuck
off'-ing thing.
There was no profit to gain from the prophet they
were proffering.

So I let in what I missed.
Felt them in the midst of my heart and the heart
of their midst.

I was open to receiving.
The reprieve of my grieving came down to
believing.
Retrieving.
Retrieving my believing was all I was needing.

Buddha, Shiva, Mohammed, Jesus, Jehovah were
all quite delighted.
I had a huge spirit party with all the gurus invited.

They understood it wasn't personal
Remaining unshakable while I was immersed
submersible
The curse that I cursed was reversed like Sir
Percival.

So I let in what I missed
Felt them in the midst of my heart, and the heart
of their midst.

My purpose was heightened
My journey's not finished but my path is
enlightened
Ignited
To brighten my light as bright as can be lightened

In shining luminous I'll start to repay for my
insolent scoff
And fall into knowledge ever solid, and a love
light ever soft.

Stepping out of the skin of the spiritual layman.
To celebrate and co-create a new age soul
relation... Amen.

Percival was laying supine on the bed, one hand on his heart, one on his stomach. His face untroubled and serene. At first Daniel was going to wake him up but he held his tongue and regarded this man that had given him so much. It was not a long time, maybe a minute or two, but in the stillness of seeing his belly slowly rising and falling, Daniel was awed, much as a parent may be in watching their own sleeping child.

And then he was hungry. For food. So he went to the kitchen and prepared himself a meal fit for someone who had just come back from a long distant inward journey around the universe. A contemplative old man gaze like something out of a 1980's instant coffee commercial was across his face as he said his grace.

... Thank you...

Two pieces of 9-grain bread with almond butter and raspberry jam slathered on top. Two eggs over-easy with pepper and a can of beans. Two quinoa flour pancakes with ghee (A clarified butter that Percival had introduced him to) and Quebec maple syrup. A shake with banana, berries, fresh coriander, bee pollen, chia seeds, spirulina, and a scoop of Vega protein powder, and finally a cup of English Breakfast tea.

All told it had taken him just over 20 minutes to prepare but it looked like a bomb had gone off in the kitchen. Around his plates though was cleared of any clutter. Every piece of the meal held its own space and had had attention put into the presentation.

Unlike the dead man walking's last meal however, Daniel felt his entire life at his feet. No thoughts as to where he was going or what he was doing, just an immense and profound rawness of love and opportunity.

… Life loves me…

Each flavour, every morsel, was like walking through an old Victorian estate mansion where each room is a world of its own. Library (Oooh a fireplace), games room (Pool table… Sweet!), bathing chamber (Look at the size of that bathtub?!), dining room (Elaborate meticulous china settings). Not to say he was dainty in the eating of it. A truck-stop cowboy was more close to the mark in terms of his etiquette. Grunting and humming his approval throughout. Huge forkfuls ballooning his cheeks. He finished it all save for some spoonfuls of beans and a quarter cup of tea. Looking around him, immensely satisfied, he simply got up and made his way back upstairs.

Stepping into the shower he let the cold water tighten up his skin and muscles. A spontaneous gasp at the shock of it and a smile at the whole body sensations.

… I won the lottery of life…

Hair and body washed he stood in front of the mirror and lathered his face. These were ablutions. The conscious ritual of cleansing and care for a body that has been entrusted to the individual. Temple, playground, machine, instrument, spaceship.

His entire form had transformed. He could see this now. Lithe and long muscles, skin a healthy glow, sharp eyes.

Walking back down to the kitchen he had designs on clearing up the mess from his meal.

"I'm leaving today Daniel." He stopped dead in his tracks. Percival stood at the sink washing the dishes.

"I was just coming to do those." An odd part of him thinking that leaving the dishes was the reason for Percival's statement.

"It's time."

"Time for what? You just said the other day that I had a lot to learn Sonny boy."

"We've done all we can to get you prepared. Me staying around for any longer will only imbue a sense of dependency. Plus..." His smile broadened. "I've got to go live my life." Percival went back to washing up. Daniel was at a loss for what to say or do. His purpose had been to wash the dishes. He hadn't put any thought beyond that. Impulsively he walked over and grabbed the broom out of the hallway closet and began to sweep the kitchen floor. He needed to do something.

"My entire purpose in coming into your life was to help you regain control of it. That's my job and gift, I'm a cleaner."

"Janitorman."

There was a slightly perceptible rise in his posture as though he had received a high compliment. "Ha ha, yeah. And now my job has come to the end of its practicality. I've really learned so much about myself and my duty. Thank you so much for your strength and perseverance throughout our time together."

"How can you be grateful to me? All I've done is taken from you."

"It would be a pretty horrible world if everyone was giving and no one received eh?"

"I guess, but…" He hung his head.

"But what?"

"I'm not ready for you go!"

"Oh Daniel… You beautiful man… I can't be the one that tells you how this story ends." It was such a tender and gentle smile that filled his entire face.

"I was thinking about how I see life. What I mean to say is that I think I can hear how it speaks to me."

Percival dried his hands on a dishtowel and sat down at the countertop.

Chapter 25: Play On

"I don't know how to play any instruments and I definitely wouldn't be able to read sheet music, but there is a melody and rhythm to my life's energy that feels like I'm in one giant musical score."

"Like Broadway?"

"Ha! Like everything. Like the Beatles, like Frank Sinatra or the Daft Punk. You had said that it was a giant lovemaking session, but I think for me it's more like an immense orchestra playing the most refined and divine opus I could imagine. Whatever is playing I feel myself to be a fluid organic instrument of it. Dancing and moving to the tempo, but at the same time I am also the beat and bass making me move." He took a deep breath, savouring the moment as words he had always known but never spoken began to formulate. "I'm singing a song and that song is me... and... and the deeper I feel it, the more I release into the creation of what wants to be sung, of what wants to be played, and of what wants to be directed or conducted in the next notes."

"Pitch perfect."

"And it's not like I'm hearing the notes being played all the time, it's more like they are resonating at different frequencies in my spine and limbs and consciousness. Sort of like... kind of like a xylophone."

"Or maybe like a reed flute?"

"Um, well that's not the first instrument to pop into my head, but yeah, I guess so." He had a vision of the Pied Piper of Hamlin dancing down the street with hordes of rats and children in tow.

"The reed flute is an allegory utilized by Rumi."

"The poet right?" Daniel had a vague recollection of hearing his name at different points in his life, but had never sought out his work.

"Not just a poet Daniel, this is a man from the 13th Century that talks across time and boundaries of space to make it feel like the words he's using are talking to you, about you, and from you all at the same time."

"Wow." Daniel was not impressed. He was just saying wow to placate Percival. He didn't want to talk about Rumi, he wanted to talk about himself. "I wrote another poem." The inflection in his voice insinuating the question 'You want to read it?'

"Awesome! I'd love to!"

"Yeah sure… But you don't have to if you don't want to."

"Daniel why do you play these silly games? There's no need to protect your self from rejection by putting in that postscript. You just put the conversation spotlight back onto yourself and then you shirk it off with a flippant offer for me to reneg on the reading of it."

Daniel started laughing and shaking his head. "God you're good man, I would be delighted if you read my poem."

"Excellent. It would be my pleasure."

Chapter 26: Dreamscape

…If only my loneliness were only less…

He was walking towards the peak of a Himalayan mountain. It was nighttime. The plateau was windswept and covered with huge snowdrifts. A solitary suburban Canadian house, brick and vinyl siding, with its lights out and curtains drawn was in shadow to the left. He walked up to the front door only to find it locked. The doorbell created no sound.

Walking over to the cliffs edge he peered down into the valley. The soft little yellow lights of a village were below, quite far below. But for some reason he felt as though he could hear the warmth and laughter emanating from the pantries and firesides. There was a longing to be in that environment even though he knew he had chosen the climb and isolation.

The crunch of snow underfoot was visceral but there was no effect of cold. A sensation of weightlessness and dis-attachment, a half lucid knowing that he was dreaming. Ssshhhkt It's one small step for man sssshhhkt… One giant leap for mankind.

Chapter 27: *In the Wake*

It was a week since Percival had packed up his bag and left. Daniel was in a confused depression mixed with bouts of nostalgic recollection and mental gymnastics. Replaying scenarios to a point of mania.

He was sick at himself for neglecting the early morning ritual that had been a mainstay for the previous three months. He hadn't done his mirror work since the last and first time, and writing was a non-starter. Hell, once again he wasn't even shaving.

The shame spiral was virulent. The more he sat around doing nothing, the more he would subjugate himself to inner admonitions of worthlessness.

… Down and down and down he goes, where he stops nobody knows…

The weather had changed in unison with his mood. Grey overcast skies and the tide of green leaves turning to autumn hues. Mont Royal was a deluge of bronze and gold. A downcast drizzling rain that keeps everyone inside except only the most ardent of dog walkers had started three days previous and hadn't stopped.

Daniel's mind was fixated on the conversation Percival and he had had before his departure. The smile, *that God damned playful smile*, imprinted on his psyche after he dropped his bombshell. "It doesn't change all the work you've done."

From the time he awoke he had been in the stupor and gravity of internet surfing. Revisiting page after page of variant monotony, his eyes were a lighter shade of glaze.

And then… sssshhkt… while sat in a pair of sweat pants surrounded by pizza boxes, bags of junk food, and a rather off putting odor, he slapped the laptop shut.

… This is another form of paralysis…

"Fuck it. I'm done." One huge breath and a sobering look around shocked him to his feet. "This is insane. Why would I want this as my life?" It was a lightning bolt of insight.

… Everything is a frequency. Light and sound waves, heat and electricity. My body and emotions. Even this God damned melancholy. My patterns of thought and the way I see the world and my place in it are frequencies. I'm transmitting a Morse code of requests and statements, why would I be surprised at the response?…

He needed a change of scenery. No time to shower, even though he had all the time in the world. Throwing on a pair of boots and a rain jacket he headed out into the wet dreary day and immediately felt better. The clack of his boots on the pavement were a reassurance. Besides a couple trips to the corner depanneur (Montreal's version of the convenience store) his activity had been largely inert. Feeling the mental haze lifting, his body was like a racehorse in the starting gates. Nostrils flaring and front hooves pawing at the ground. His body was ready to RUN.

What few people he did cross, he wanted to connect with them. Holding back the compulsion to run over and give them a hug.

He started to walk faster. No idea where he was going, that was the last of his concerns. Because he was the force propelling himself forwards. This wasn't doing what he had done before, stuck in the conventional consumerism and dictates of a dead end job. Nor was it follow the leader, like with Percival. He was the leader, and the pride and autonomy he felt was, well, it was liberating.

By the time he got to St. Laurent he knew exactly where he was headed.

When he first arrived in Montreal, one of the first things he had done was walk to the top of Mont Royal. That was close to 6 years ago, and the novelty had worn off in the first ascension.

The statutes of the city state that no building can exceed the height of the mountain. With its radio tower and giant crucifix, the mountain is the heart of the city. The downtown business core may be its brain, the old port its lungs, and the plateau area its stomach, but the mountain itself was the heart and soul of all that surrounded it. Looking down on the city and beyond from the observation deck one can see the metropolis in a different light. Other mountains on the distant horizon, like self proclaimed watchmen, call back with their presence. The St. Lawrence River separating the island from the mainland and bridges of various sizes along the shores stitched the two together. The perpetual movements and activities of a 3.5 million populace walking, biking, and driving.

He was walking up Avenue des Pins towards McGill University. A parade of colourful umbrellas now on either side of the street. Because, while people for the most part will wear black and grey clothing, they allow themselves the luxury of a splash of colour or pattern in their parapluie. Up along Dr. Penfield Drive, past the Royal Victoria Hospital, brought him to a set of wooden stairs leading up the side of his destination. He ascended them two at a time. The stairs themselves only led about a quarter of the way up. A winding back and forth path along the face was carved up the rest of the way. Daniel didn't want to take that option. He picked a line straight through the brush and rocks. Scrambled through the 25 or 30 feet until the next platform and then set another line straight up. The ground was slick.

His hands were covered in earth and bits of foliage from trying to prevent a major fall. A stupid smile on his reddening face and heavy strong breaths. Up to the third or fourth step his right foot slipped out behind him and he fell onto his left side. His knee made an audible thump on a protruding root. The laugh and yelp came out simultaneously.

"H-ow-ly fuck! Oh my god! Hoooo that hurt." Shaking it off he made the final face. This one reminded him of a rampart of a castle. More rocky and vertical than the others, there was of course the path leading off to the left around the top, but there was no question.

Getting to the top he was a soaking mess. Sweat pants were definitely the wrong selection, and his rain shell, while preventing the rain from getting in, was holding in the humidity and heat of his body ensuring that he was sweating like a beast.

…Jesus I'm hot…

The view was better than he remembered. Looking to the east he could see the giant green blue arches of the Jacques Cartier Bridge, and all the way west of that, through downtown, Westmount, Verdun and Lasalle, and into the

West Island. Heart pounding in his chest his breaths were still heaving. Coming to a standstill the next wave of heat rolled through him.

… I'm roasting!…

Unzipping his jacket and unhooking the Velcro cuffs he simply let the jacket drop to the ground. Cotton t-shirt clinging to him in a heavy steaming mass.

Chapter 28: The Good-Bye

They were stood at the platform of Mont Royal metro station. Had been for the past four trains. It was mainly Percival who was speaking. Daniel walking beside at a slightly slower pace, eyes downcast, with the look of a child not wanting his favourite summer camp to come to an end. That was until Percival let slip the little tidbit that Daniel had been reeling over in his isolation for the past week.

"Wait… What did you just say?"

Now it might seem funny to most, or even all, but Daniel had not really questioned why Percival had knocked on his door in the first place. In fact he had almost built up a magical fairytale-like blind spot around it all. The way things had unfolded, and the complete presence that Percival had shown at every corner made it seem… destined.

"I was just laughing about some of the other responses I got from the doors I knocked on before yours. There was this one francophone mother with two young kids that…"

"But you said that you came to me because I asked for a teacher?"

"I did. And you did."

"But you were at other houses first?"

"Yeah, a lot of them. Ten at least." He was chuckling and shaking his head at the memory. "And you just can't go door to door knocking at peoples houses telling them you're their teacher. You'd get arrested for sure."

"This is crazy."

"Tell me about it. That's why after knocking at one house I'd go to an entirely different part of town. Verdun, Westmount, Ahuntsic."

"But, but, you knew my name!?"

"Yeah that was funny wasn't it? I had just watched 'Karate Kid' the week before and I was feeling all Mr. Myagi." Wax on, wax off hands. "It was one of those wonderful coincidences we've had so often."

"Why didn't you tell me that at the time?"

"Because the mystery and random nature of that moment ensured a stronger foothold to work with you. Imagine if I had said that I had no idea who you were at the time? I wasn't talking to Daniel Shaughnessy, I was talking to the humanity of you."

"I feel like you cheated on me."

"Well I feel like you're not very appreciative of all that I've done for you in the past three months. My perspective was much larger at the time. Those others weren't ready to listen to what I had to say. For whatever reason they weren't ready. You were, you chose the wake-up call."

"You lied to me though. You led me on."

"You selfish shit. Why don't you think of someone else for once? Do you know how incredibly difficult and vulnerable it is to audaciously walk up to an absolute stranger and talk to a piece of them that in most cases is neglected and forlorn? To be given guarded looks of mistrust and fear when offering your best love and purity? It's heartbreaking."

For the first time ever Daniel saw a depth of sadness in Percival that scared him.

... *Mine would say 'Please love me'...*

"But I can't let that stop me giving my gift Daniel. Me coming to you was coincidence, yes, but it was also too random to be anything else other than divine. And so that is not coincidence any longer. It's divinity. It's life loving itself. But it was also me trying to honour my heart song. Honour my gifts and my place in the world. I didn't come here for you…" Cue the Cobra Kai 'Sweep the leg' phrase. "…I came here for me."

Another train going towards Cote Vertu pulled into the platform. Daniel made eye contact with the driver as the head of the train streamed past. The noise gave them both a chance to pause.

… So what does this mean to me? Where does it leave me?…

An illusion of innocence was broken for Daniel in that moment. The Wizard of Oz curtain was pulled aside to reveal what his wild flailing thoughts had said in their first encounter. He needed some time and space to process this, but he also knew that any time and space taken now would be permanent.

… I'm not special to him at all…

His decision to walk away at that moment was made to show how strong and independent he was. And however much that might have been true to him, the 1 or 2% inside of him that was turning away in spite, was the major factor in his downward spiral in the week following.

"I was trying to create a language from a space that I've only known internally." Percival's voice was growing to coincide with the gap between them widening. "In the expression externally comes more understanding of those things not of this world." Crossing the bridge across the tracks towards the exit were the last words Daniel would hear him speak. "It doesn't change all the work you've done!"

… I've abandoned my love…

Chapter 27(a): **In the Wake**

Old habits die hard. It's not like the water of thought just, all of the sudden, up and decides to flow in a different direction.

Standing at the top of the island, all water runs downhill.

Daniel's relationships had one seemingly constant theme. Abandon or be abandoned. At some point the depth or intensity would touch the sensitive sacred wound and create the same patterned protective response.

The drizzle that had been continuous for the past three days was increasing. The fine mist was turning into big droplets. Matted hair was directing streams down his forehead and cascading over the features of his face. Water ran down his jaw line to the point of his chin.

It was beautiful. All around him puddles were splashed with a million billion raindrops. His heart swelled with the blessings of all that he had, and the absolute abundance that surrounded him. He was a blessillionaire.

… Of the 3.5 million people in this city I'm the only one here right now…

The giggles started as the perfection of the sounds all around permeated his being. Taking his shirt off, his bare torso and nervous system ignited in sensual awareness. Each drop and rivulet sending messages to his brain, and the brain, in kind, sent its own information response back. The spider at the centre of the spider web. Arms moved effortlessly into outstretched reaching. Eyes closed and face turned towards to the sky. Music was everywhere. It was everything.

This was freedom. This was full expression. There's the point when you get so wet, or so dirty that it literally doesn't matter how much more wet or dirty you get.

As a drunken 23 year-old Daniel had turned his face to the sky and yelled as loud as he could "FUCK YOU!" The university friends that were with him at the dead of night went stock still and silent. The outburst had come from out of nowhere and was directed upwards. Daniel didn't even really know where it had come from. There was a piece of him that obviously felt like it was getting a raw deal. He didn't quite know who or what he was shouting out, but something changed for him at that moment. It was the beginning and the end of his victim. Rage and confusion had sewn a seed in his garden. And it was the presence of this foreign eyesore that was, in an unconscious way, the reason for Daniel's readiness (eagerness?) to welcome Percival across his threshold. While he didn't have the words or wisdom at the time to even know what was wrong with his life, the baobab had gestated to a big enough degree to have created his exasperated plea 'Oh God, Why can't this all just cease?'

Standing and laughing in the rain now, because not only did he see the perfection of where he was in this moment, topless and hysterically happy, but he saw the perfection of that rage and confusion. He saw its absolute necessity and the role of that bitterness as a young man to bring him to this point.

… Never underestimate the power of a horrible example…

The same entity of life he had sworn off as an immature man-boy, was the same entity that brought a saving grace in the form of a young blonde-haired, blue-eyed... Yes, I feel he was that to me if to no one else... Angel.

The same dysfunction had produced the penicillin antidote to its corruption and left the forged ingot of wisdom and experience in its wake. His heart, whispering sweet nothings, was telling its own story to itself.

"Excusez-moi, est ce que ca va?" (Excuse me, is everything alright?)

A man in his mid-60's, with a huge golf umbrella and soaking wet Labrador stood a few feet behind him.

Turning from his reverie with no guard or resistance in place, no thought pollution, they made eye contact. The expression on the man's face changed from questioning concern to one of surprise instantly.

...Mon dieu, ses yeux sont tellement claire... (My god, his eyes are so clear)

"Oui... oui merci. Tout va bien. Il fait parfait aujourd'hui." (Yes... Yes thank you. Everything is fine. It's perfect today.)

The dog took one step forward and the master one step back.

"Uhhh, ben oui, donc... bonne journee." (Uh, good well, so... have a good day.)

"Merci monsieur, et vous aussi." (Thank you sir, and you also)

Daniel reached down and picked up his jacket, shaking it a few times before putting it back on. He held his sopping shirt in his right hand and took one last long panoramic gaze around him. His body was shivering with a chill. With no wallet, no phone, and no problem with that, he started back home and a hot shower. He'd take the path down this time.

Chapter 29: **Pearls of Wisdom**

"Do you know how a pearl is created?"

Since getting back from the mountain the day before, Daniel had reestablished his routine. Early morning rise and shine, triple 'S', meditation, hot lemon and water, and then a yoga practice. By the time all was said and done it was just past 8:30. So our intrepid hero did what any self-respecting unemployed man in this situation would do. He went out for a coffee and a pastry.

Which brought him to a high dark wooden table top in Olive & Gourmando. A patisserie café in the heart of the Old Port that oozes the French sensibilities of rich baked goods and wild gesticulating conversation. The man standing beside him was a character no doubt. Salt and pepper Mohawk, and a perfectly crafted handlebar moustache with lightning bolt sideburns dyed jet black. Snakeskin boots and strong musk cologne. The eccentricity of this man would stand out anywhere, but at quarter past 9 in the morning, it was too blatant for Daniel to avoid or ignore such a direct conversation starter.

"You mean besides the fact that an oyster makes it?"

"It starts off as an irritant, a piece of sand let's say, and…" The dark haired waitress placed a small espresso cup and saucer down for the man, and carried away two empty ones that were in front of him. He gave her a fast smile and then winked at Daniel, taking an inrush of breath to create a slight whistling sound. It was a playful action, nothing leering or creepy in the delivery. "… and gradually gets coated to protect and soothe the inhabitant of the shell. The oyster takes something annoying and turns it into something precious. All it needs is a little time." Saying that he picked up his espresso, downed it in one shot, and then stood up to leave.

… I guess that's all he had to say about that. (A la Forrest Gump)…

"Uh, thanks." Daniel was a little bit stunned. He felt as though he was just given a pearl of his own. And as quickly as it was given, the one who had bestowed the gift, stood up and walked away. No muss, no fuss.

His own Americano and brioche arrived as the plodding clop-clop of a horse drawn carriage ricocheted on the cobbles and facades of rue St. Paul outside. It was a quick grace he gave before eating. Not only did it slow everything down, but it gave him a slight giddy anticipation about the fact that he got to eat the beautiful food placed before him in the first place. Taking a whistling breath of his own, after the first bite of dark chocolate and pecan brioche. Buttery, warm and moist goodness.

An atmosphere of laughter and loud talking surrounded him. Bustling waitresses laden with plates going to bustling tables exuding the Gallic tendency of joie de vie. Eating, talking and making merry. Bustling businessmen and women picking up their to-go coffee and little brown bag treat from the bustling baristas. The lovely thing was that though he was by himself it did not feel awkward. If a person looked over in his direction, more often than not Daniel found they would exchange a slight smile of acknowledgment. Much of the commotion of the room centered around the pastry counter that doubled as the cashier. Plates of piled high delicacies all with their own special allure. Daniel was certain that the baked goods heightened the happiness factor of all those present. It was that thought, like music to his ears, that kept him so content.

... Everyone seems so content...

Percival had something when he spoke of his gift. It was a solidity that seemed to have the world revolve around his axis. No matter what he was talking about it felt as though he was grounded and rooted in his speech. Daniel thought back to his first mirror working session, how never in a million years would he have done something like that even a few months prior, and yet after firm direction, he stepped right into it. Percival stated, by his presence alone, "This is how we do it."

... I wonder what my gift is?...

This question had been niggling for weeks. Going through life without purpose is like forever walking around a junior high dance floor without a partner. Rather than the comfort and security of belonging, hands on the girl's hips, swaying side to side to Boyz II Men, there is the isolation and discomfort of not really having 'fit' anywhere. Hands are jammed in pockets, shoulders shrugged up to the ears, and a not so subtle wanting to be someone, anyone, else.

Of course the adolescent need to find that partner is a form of protection and conformity, whereas the adult's direction is to honour and express the gift almost in spite of comfort or safety. Artists know this. We sacrifice our comfort in order to unearth the gift. We sacrifice our life story to develop and refine the gift. We sacrifice past stages of conformity to bare ourselves raw and vulnerable to the world.

Breaking free from those bonds can be devastating to one uninitiated internally because without 100% certainty, without full faith, self-doubt can spread like a plague to the very roots of one's own passion.

Percival had that certainty. He held mastery of his craft.

… Fuck was he ever proud of being a cleaner…

"So you don't have any apple turnovers?" Even the constant din of the café could not muffle the grating nasally voice at the counter.

"No madam, everyt'ing we 'ave is 'ere." The cashier's voice was heavily laden with French.

"Everything is here?"

The cannonball from daydreaming to judging would give an F1 driver whiplash. Five things flashed through Daniel's mind in quick rapid fire.

1. They're called chaussons aux pommes here bitch!
2. Yes! That's what she said. Can't you understand English?
3. God her voice is so irritating.
4. Percival's voice saying "When you stop thinking about how something is "supposed" to be, and start seeing it for what it actually is, that is the moment you will feel happiness in the form of perfection.
5. Everything is here for you…

That fifth phrase kept repeating itself over and over in his head. Multiple voices and degrees of authority all touching upon a secret code locked away in some recess. There was nothing urgent in the unfolding. More like a curiosity and awe when seeing a 3D image pop off a page for the first time. The visual stimulus of the café, along with the external sounds and smells were melding into his thoughts and stream of consciousness. Touching a key in his mind created ripples externally. A peel of laughter, someone sneezing or a synchronistic song line that made it all seem scripted. Each microscopic flutter butterfly effecting the passageway he mentally followed.

…Everything is here for me…

Not that the Maya would give up the illusion of her separateness so easily. She is an immensely intriguing enigma to elaborate. The playfulness of life increased its malleability. Down the rabbit hole of thoughts, feelings, sensations, mathematics, symbols, symbols within symbols. Hieroglyphs of a timeless soul-spell waiting to be decrypted. Daniel was playing his consciousness instrument and she danced for him. She was singing a divine aria, that at the seat of his heart, he listened to in rapture. The painter and the painting. Which was which?

… Down and down and down he goes…

Three brown paper napkins were scribbled upon. A mad collection of words and phrases came together littered with arrows, scratches and circles. A ballad to an archetype. The chords of an unknown lover.

> *I'm not standing here because I'm lost.*
> *I'm not hanging around because I'm lazy.*
> *This isn't a case of wires getting crossed.*
> *Because you are so perfectly amazingly crazy.*

This You and I mating dance.
Frantically flailing my limbs for the chance.
To glimpse your soul. Hypnotic trance.

Can't speak. Knees are weak.
It's not gushing because I'm weak.
I'm not blushing from wearing paisley.
This isn't a fashion faux pas de chic.
Because you are so perfectly amazingly crazy.

This You and I umbilical.
Tethered together in a push for the pinnacle.
A union combined, spoken, one syllable.

Oh God. Oh Lord.
I'm not climbing because I'm bored.
I'm not seeking because I'm hazy.
This isn't a fruitless search with the hoard.
Because you are so perfectly amazingly crazy.

This You and I cosmic collision.
Explosion super nova, nuclear fission.
It's ok. I'LL order our food...uhm...with your
*   permission.*

Our chariot awaits.
This is one of my most redeeming character traits.
Counting out life's blessings from A to Z.
For you they'd have to create quadruple triple 'A',
*   7 star rates.*
Because you are so perfectly amazingly crazy.

This You and I dynamite.
Your voice in my ear makes me certain it's right.
My airport fantasy, layover to flight.

Pacific ocean.
It's a sliding scale of love and devotion.
Bill Withers, Bono, Leonard Cohen and an early
*   Jay-Zee.*
It's the notion of my groove motion.
Because you are so perfectly amazingly crazy.

This You and I enormous.
Gigantic superstars in our own personal chorus.
A Cancer/Scorpio love, charging like a Taurus.

The kingdom and the glory.
When I'm writing our story.
From conception to birth to pushing up daisies.
We are living the fairytale, no worry.
Because you are so perfectly amazingly crazy.

This you and I biographic.
Opening our minds to a power telepathic.
Mind/body/soul connection. Tantric. Pornographic.

Love infusion.
I'm not writing this from a state confusion.
It took your goddess touch to raise me.
Of this there is no illusion.
You ARE perfectly amazingly crazy.
This You and I unbroken.

These thoughts and their words are but a pittance
and a token.

For a perfectly amazingly crazy woman,
indescribable, undefinable and unspoken.

CHAPTER 30: Love. Persuasion is Better Than Force

There is no definitive plan for love. No guaranteed recipe that works every time. That's the beauty of it. Daniel had no clear idea what his writing was leading him to, nor did he fully comprehend exactly where it originated, but somewhere between the future projection of where he was going (goals, expectations, dreams) and the past reflection of where he had been (stories, habits, patterns) was a pocket of beautiful and delicate creation. A bubble of insulated calm. It was an innocent space that kept hearkening to childhood times. The difference that he felt was that, as a child, he was innocent because that's what he was. Now however, that quality of innocence was bolstered by wisdom as to the value and reverence of such a state. The fragility of such beauty requires wise stewardship. Having been catapulted out of Eden, he was now finding his own passage back with gifts and experience in tow, and felt like he could make Eden a better place.

Daniel looked up from his napkins and filled his lungs to satisfaction. The long passive exhale that followed brought the underside of all supported bodily structures (bum, feet, elbows, forearms, thighs) sinking into whatever it was that held them up. It was 10:30am.

He folded up his newest poem, deposited it in his pocket, paid for his bill and walked back out into the day.

To say that it was a perfect autumn day would be an understatement. The sun was delicious while the breeze gave just a hint of cool. The spectrum of clothing that people were wearing showed the benevolence of the weather to make everyone comfortable.

… Persuasion is better than force…

Anything from a guy in a pair of shorts, topless and barefoot chasing a Frisbee, to the young professional couple walking in jeans and that favourite heavy knit sweater. The two year old waddling in front of them, colour coordinated with her mother, sporting a touque to boot. Daniel himself was in a pair of light khaki pants and a thin long sleeve.

The one consistent trait was that everyone had sunglasses on. Sunglasses and that slight unconscious upward tilt of the chin, Mona Lisa smiles, getting every ray of sunshine possible.

Daniel walked down rue St. Pierre that ends at the promenade along the Old Port quays. A mile long national park giving host to exhibitions, park benches, and a swath of casual runners. Rue de la Commune which runs parallel has an abundance of tourist boutiques, ice creams shops and hotels.

The sun was blindingly brilliant off the water. A giant red container ship named the Birchglen was moored to the stone pillared dock. Rising high above even the promenade.

Standing at the waist high round railings, Daniel scanned the length of the port. On the far side lay the Biodome and Habitat 67. The first being an Epcot-like dome, and the latter built for the World's Expo in 1967. It was a marvel of space and architecture. Distinct like a Lego building surrounded by sand castles. As he looked to his right a giant wall of silos extended down towards, what at night, was the flashing "Farine Five Roses" neon. Huddled amidst these behemoths was a black ferry boat with white lettering stenciled on its hull "Bota Bota: Spa sur L'eau"

… Go there!…

White robed individuals with hoods pulled over their heads like Jedis walked on the deck, disrobed, and stepped into a huge hot tub at the front of the foredeck. The hesitation that he had no swim trunks was met with a stern and concise order.

… Go. There. Now…

The beautiful thing about being on your own, is that the avenues of thought at one's disposal can be limitless. Explored to the very -enth degree without any need to get back to square one in order to explain or justify the rambling thoughts to another. Guided only by shifting feelings, drifting through an interior landscape of psychological cartography. In childhood it's an escape into imagination, in adulthood it takes on a Hansel and Gretel breadcrumb trail back into the imaginative freedom of those whimsical daydreams.

Daniel's thoughts had started at a distinct place, and as his feet led him forward, his thoughts wended inwardly. Broad sure-footed thoughts stepped off into smaller limbs. Long held belief structures, rocked to their foundations in the past months, were deconstructed to reveal a substratum. Which was then dissected into more intricate branches.

Whatever it was that was driving him over the loch and around the path to the spa, it was a physical rendition of a mental journey.

A CN Rail engine rumbled from in front of the silos across a bridge moving deeper into the old port. Cars laden with huge sea containers destined no doubt for spaces on ships like the Birchglen. With the distinct screech of its wheels filling the air, the weight of the train over his head could be felt in his feet.

The park to the right of the path was lush yet simply designed. Small trees and bushes surrounding a green space. On one end the rails and bridge of the CN Line, and on the other a constructed fountain and deck chairs overlooking the gangplank to the boat.

The abbreviated version of the spa visit was, buy shorts, lounge for 2 ½ hours in numerous forms of repose (Falling asleep once in a giant bean bag chair), get changed, go home. To revisit and reiterate the phrase from Percival's 22-hour span of awaiting Daniel's return however, infinite, immortal, immutable and eternal, silence and stillness is a vast land to explore.

Chapter 31: So Bota

The body works hard in a sauna or steam room. It might be relaxing and completely enjoyable to plunk down in a hot tub, but to keep the body regulated in higher temperatures is intense work.

There is something exquisitely satisfying about taking off a comfy terry towel robe and walking into a dimly lit steam room. The skin immediately sensing the change in humidity and atmospheric pressure responds with a luster of sweat. Deep full breaths expand the sinus cavity with the help of eucalyptus floating in the steam.

Silent, save for the hissing of the pipes, Daniel was the only one in the tiled circular room. The foreign feeling of his new shorts mixed with the delight to have gotten them in the first place. Clouds of steam wafted and swirled around the soft lights installed in the ceiling. Closing his eyes he leaned his head against the wall and let the heat soak into his muscles.

...Nowhere to be, nothing to do...

It hadn't even been three minutes and Daniel was dripping with sweat. Breathing through the nose at first, that slowly gave way to inhaling through the nose and exhaling out of the mouth, until after about ten minutes he was full on mouth breathing. A posture that had started out rather proud, gradually, after ten or fifteen minutes, wilted to a drooping head through the knees. Stepping up to walk out the heat on his skin increased with each movement. Leaning into the heavy glass door he stepped into the clean cool air. Lifting up his robe he noticed gold embroidery stating 'Peignoir No. 453' on the left hand sleeve.

… I am Number 453…

Red-faced and content he bowed his head to the water fountain and counted off the number of swallows he took. A little obsessive-compulsive trait having him take gulps in multiples of five.

Hood over his head, hands in his pockets, he made his way to the front sundeck and a date with a hot tub.

The vieux port promenade, heavily populated with pedestrians, bicycles, strollers, and a small army of joggers was confronted by the Old World mystique of 18th Century architecture. Contrasting that, the modern skyline of downtown Montreal rose behind in New World efficiency. An exquisite panorama postcard at the worst of times, to be sitting in a giant shamrock shaped hot tub on top of a boat is to get actively absorbed into the postcard.

A flat metal question mark on the bow of the ship arced a hot sheet of water back into the tub. Two couples and a small group of three sat at different points talking or giggling in hushed tones.

Daniel situated himself in the sunshine with a view of the promenade. A jet massaged his back. Closing his eyes and leaning his head back, the smile on his face would have been comical if it wasn't so genuine. A game show host called Wink Binkleman would be proud of such a smile "Tell him what he's won Bob!"

Numerous people stop to take photos of Bota Bota. As though with that photo they can say they have been somewhere or experienced something vicariously through the faceless bodies that litter the decks. The concept of luxury being a chasm too great to span. Self-worth, when it comes to such blatant (Yet soooooo necessary) decadence is not as easy to justify as an unselfish act costing the same amount of money for someone else.

Daniel was definitely not thinking about money. Or the fact that he was jobless and slapped with a reputation placed squarely in the shitter. His lifeboat was rudderless and for now, as stupid as it may sound, it felt like everything was exactly as it should be.

People floated through his head. Percival, Melanie and past lovers, Jared and Dick LePage. The relationships he shared and how they reflected back to him his own virtues and deficiencies. He saw his Self, immature, and then slightly less immature, after each tryst and intimate encounter. Because no matter how hard one might try to protect the heart with self-proclamations of "I don't care" or "It's not a big deal" being naked in the arms of another will cut to the raw and show where love is lacking. These visions of impotence for a man-boy are designed to destroy what is limiting said man-boy from evolving into that beautiful and strong space of manhood. Full bodied, erect and proud. No matter the situation, a gentleman does the job to his absolute and most honest effort because that is the purpose. The gift is the work. The outcome is what can be gifted or bestowed as suited, but an oyster doesn't make the pearl with the idea to give it away.

Daniel could see that those women who had shared his bed had also challenged him to be a better man. They filled his heart with a medicine that stung to the core, but also gave solutions to the pain.

He could see his tendency and addiction to that love angst because it let him know he was alive. Just like the pain response in the human body lets the entire form know of a burnt finger, Daniel had perpetuated his dysfunction in order to (Crazy I know) feel his existence. As though by bearing the weight of suffering and dragging the misery along he was paying for his life.

… No one's interested in something you didn't do…

His own story was separate from him. Sitting in the audience, he watched memories and cameo appearances alight his stage.

Imagine me. Before creation. Before being created. And now imagine me, as I am, stepping into the lone spotlight on an otherwise darkened stage. Somehow, magically, full of form and character. 31 years appearing to you as one moment. It's not so far fetched.

Who would play me in the story of me? Who would play Daniel Shaughnessy in the story of Daniel Shaughnessy? I've been doing it my whole life, but perhaps my contract has expired, or the production company wants to take another direction. The executive producer has had enough and he says "Who else can we get to play this Shaughnessy guy?" Pressing the intercom on his desk he moves his face closer to the receiver and commands "Janice, get me a list of some casting agencies pronto." There'd only be a second pause before a sharp voice would come back in reply, "Yes sir. Right away Mr. Executive Producer." Because, even though she's worked for him for just over three decades, he demands that he be referred to by his title. She is Janice.

As a long running tragicomedy the director and stagehands are seasoned professionals. Cameo characters and guest appearances have come and gone. The one protagonist that the audience has ever known has just, unknown to him, played his last role as the intrepid hero. Now how does this executive break the news to the kid who he, and millions of others, have watched grow from a child into a man playing this role of one Daniel Michael Shaughnessy?

"Daniel…it's really hard to tell you this…Aww geez, this is the toughest part of my job…Dan… did you ever have a hamster as a kid?…"

This new actor would bring his own spin to the role. Maybe play it a bit more edgy. Be the bad boy persona. Wearing more black and placing expletives into normal everyday conversation "This is some good fxxxing pad thai."

He would say, "I think Daniel would be a smoker", and so now I have a pack of smokes in my pocket along with a can of Binaca spray. As much as I'd be a bad ass, I'd still be conscious of bad breath.

"…What I mean to say, Daniel, is that…well… you've been with us a long time. You've been loyal to us. Even in the hard times. In the lean times. You've been there through it all. Hey you remember that time when you went on that camping trip and you fell off that cliff into the waterfall? And then the current pulled you over the cascades?! Man, we all thought you were a goner…"

Would this new guy make deeper advancements in my life? Write the book I'd always felt was within me. Be mature and responsible enough to own a plant or two? It'd be tough to watch someone make better and more efficient use of the time given to him. To watch them be, for lack of a better term, a better human. A better Daniel Shaughnessy. A better me. Because what is it to be human if it is not to create? To make something, where before there was nothing. Placing your Self in the inferno of failure and coming out the other end with a forged ingot. The placement of time, energy, and intention into something uncertain. It took Michaelangelo 4 years to paint the Sistine Chapel. 4 Years!!! Imagine the learning curve of the Self in such focus.

"…Basically, what it is coming down to is numbers…"

Not to say that a new actor coming into this character would find it easy or seamless. As much as it's a simple life, it's not always easy. There's a lot of intangibles to be taken care of. And viewers might grow suspect if the preparations had not been made. Envision the middle-aged housewife, head poking around the corner, curlers in the hair, bathrobe a worn shade of burgundy, the giant wooden spoon covered with spaghetti sauce in her right hand "Honey?! Didn't Daniel used to be able to make that high pitched whistle between his teeth?"

Back to the executive producer breaking the news, "… You know some of the best things in my life have come out of a major ending. I never would have met my wife if I didn't get in that car accident a few years back for example. You should have seen her face at the time, it was priceless…"

An actor always wants to have the big role. Which makes me wonder if they would cross boundaries of inner moral truths to play another character? Would one be able to justify their actions in the name of another?

Which is sort of what defense attorneys do. "It wasn't HIM, your Honour, it was another, crazy, maniacal "him". So don't punish the him that is in fact him for the "him" that was not him when it was that other "him" that was not him who did it. The defense rests." What sort of compromises have some made in their line of work? In their line of life?

Back to the company exec "…and you'll always be the original Daniel Shaughnessy, Daniel, no one can take that away from you…"

Sitting in that office. Listening to the executive say anything and everything, except what needs to be said. Trying to soften the blow when, in fact, nothing needs to be softened. I gave my best to the role, and now it's time to move on. The need to BE someone fades. It's an evolution to a new phase of my life… whatever, and whomever, that might be.

It would be the old cliché, years from now, to have someone come up to me in a coffee shop or supermarket "Hey?! Aren't you Daniel Shaughnessy?!" Face wrinkled and unshaven. Dressed in an unassuming manner. Still with a trace of the old flash and flare in my eyes, "I used to be kid…I used to be."

Start all over. Starting from scratch is a new beginning.

Opening his eyes Daniel rose from his submerged seat and stepped out into the brisk cool air. His whole body alive and titillated. Wrapping up in his robe, he stepped back into the spa for another round at the water fountain. Ten sips. Licking his lips and taking a survey of his surroundings he started towards the sauna on the starboard side. Entering the dry cedar heat, the air was distinctly tinted with lemon. A bank of bench seats covered the left side of the room, while the right side wall was floor to ceiling windows looking out onto the port and the huge red hull of the Birchglen. Three stands of dry rocks with two wooden buckets, ladles included, were filled with water and a film of oil that was no doubt the source of the citrus scent.

One man, lying supine with an arm across his face, was on the top tier. The hourglass on the wall was marking at five minutes. Daniel sat himself at the other side of the room on the middle level. Hands on his knees and feet squarely placed onto the planks of the lowest bench.

Staring at the port was hypnotizing. The canvas of the waters surface responded and then absorbed the invisible movements of the wind. Midday in the middle of Montreal and other than his sweating companion there was not a soul in sight. Coming into stillness Daniel began to see not only how much movement there was, but also how much was immobile. Internally was the same paradox, immense stillness with fluid expression.

Hypersensitive from the heat, trickles of sweat massaged their way down his body. Rivulets taking on a venous movement. Unlike the steam room his posture was actually growing through the intensity. The man beside him gave a grunt and then sat up.

"Ca vous derange si je place plus d'eau sur les roches?" (Will it bother you if I put more water on the rocks?) His voice was a deep and gravelly bass. The question caught Daniel a touch off guard and brought him from his reverie.

… Holy shit, he wants it hotter?…

"Non, non, vas-y." (No, no go ahead)

The searing hiss of the water hitting the rocks and the subsequent wafts of heat shocked him into a new headspace. In a word, the best way to describe it would be competitive. As though, because the man was in the room before he was, he should leave first.

Never mind the fact that the survivalist instinct had alarm bells ringing. Being pressed to the limit physically allows us to see where the cracks are. Anyone can retain composure when life's element is on simmer, but turn the notch up to high and inconsistencies will present themselves in pretty quick succession.

The 15-minutes of the hourglass sand had run out while the man ladled water onto the rocks.

…Why don't you just pour the whole bucket on there asshole?!...

Putting the ladle back in the bucket the man casually flipped the hourglass and went back to his spot.

Daniel's whole body was in overdrive. The heat was everywhere but seemed to specifically centre in his head. Blood pressure absolutely throbbing in his temples.

… Well he's lying down, that's why he's not freaking out…

Each excuse as to why this man could stay in the sauna longer than Daniel was met with an argument on the other side, which just incensed the aggravation.

… He's been in here 5 minutes longer than you have…

… He has a towel to lie on, I don't have a towel…

… Yes but he's on the upper tier and you're only on the second…

… He's intentionally doing this to fuck with me…

… Yeah, well, maybe he is…

… OK, 10 more seconds and then I am out of here. 10, 9, 8, 7, 6, 5, urgh I'm serious, 4, 3, 2, 1, …

He pressed into his hands to stand up. It had been another five minutes of sand falling in slow motion. His skull felt like a hammer was hitting it. Pressing into the glass door, the magnet disengaged, and the sweet blessed breathable air was salvation to a taxed nervous system. The cold tub in front of him promised too convenient a respite to pass up so he stepped into the 4C water and immediately felt the vasoconstriction of every blood vessel in contact. Up to his crotch in freezing water, the muscles tightened and the breath was spasmodic and shallow. Garnering his courage he sat down so only his head and neck were above the meniscus of the waterline.

Daniel felt the cold tub like sharp glass. Funny how in that moment he compared the different viscosities of the hydrotherapies he had done. The heat of the steam room felt like a soft and warm 3-dimensional embrace. The hot tub was a white molten bubbly heat, while the sauna was dry unforgiving prairie fire. Each one had its own qualities to experience or learn from.

… Everything is a frequency. I've been bathing myself in different levels of light and experience, like moving from one aquarium to another…

Taking a big inhalation and holding his breath, he submerged himself. It was actually easier to be fully underwater. The body was still cold, but in a way it was comforting to feel the uniformity. Any heat tension was emanating out, while feelings of tingling and cleansing washed over his form. A vision of the port's water surface responding to the gusting north winds flashed in his mind.

Getting out of the tub he wrapped up in his robe, walked to one of the giant beanbag chairs, and sunk into a state of grace. If indeed he had gone into four different aquariums of varying pressure or intensity, his nervous system was now completely happy to drop into a phase where it was unchallenged and able to find a natural state of equilibrium. Wrapped from tip to tail in his towel and robe, arms nestled into the sleeves of the opposite arm, and hood covering his face, there was not one patch of skin visible. In the cocoon of white terry cloth Daniel sunk into an interstitial layer between waking and sleeping.

The decryption of patterns and spoon fed "truths" happens in this space. A release from identification allows for the new code to be written. Where there was once a subtle 'No' is now replaced by a wise 'Yes'.

In the very early formative years of life, from 0-2 years of age, there is little to no verbal language. An infant is so beautifully at the mercy of the environment that it needs to surrender fully and wholly to survive. As the individual grows it's easy to learn how to take care of oneself physically (Brushing teeth, wiping the bum) and intellectually (reply to an email, pay a bill) but when it comes to being emotionally independent, many individuals are still reliant on exterior sources of love and attention to give them a sense of nourishment. Growing out of emotional infancy, childhood, or adolescence and becoming a smart and self-activated human being (as opposed to a reactive human animal) is the invisible obstacle facing most modern "adults". Having not yet flipped the switch to feel an inward wellspring to be the primary source of love and light for the Self, each person is either consciously or unconsciously dissatisfied. Instead of listening to their own essential and inherent intelligence, they have given over this birthright to the dictates of parental, societal, or dogmatic beliefs as to what the individual should be or do.

The generational axiom for Daniel's parents would be "Out of sight, out of mind." Because they had the luxury of dumping shit, literally and figuratively, and not seeing the repercussions. Ignoring something was a completely viable option. As the world shrinks the reverberation of consequences can be almost immediate. Responsibility and integrity are tantamount. The anesthesia of ignorance cannot cover up the dysfunction any longer.

In the primordial space, verbal language does not correlate. Truth is not housed in a word. The subconscious is not a mental construct.

The character from Olive + Gourmando popped into his head. The authenticity of how the man presented himself. In that 5-minute exchange Daniel could see that an entire encyclopedia could be written about his life and experiences. And in the enormity of the man's volume, Daniel would play a miniature part on one of the pages.

... From beginning to end, I see it...

He opened his eyes and took his first inhale. The sanity and cleanliness of his mind left no doubt as to the next step. Certainty is the divine gift of purpose.

... 'Cause that's how we do it...

An hour and a half had passed by. This was an entirely different world. Daniel felt inserted into another timeline of a parallel universe. Striding to the change rooms, he was a man on a mission.

CHAPTER 32: Chapter 1

Walking through the red door he went straight to his laptop and opened a new page. Taking a deep breath, for one eternal moment, his fingers hovered above the keyboard. As a smile crossed his face, his fingers started typing.

Ding Dong.
There was the customary 30-second pause that comes after the doorbell rings. Then the vibrations and shift in air pressure as the occupant comes to unlatch the lock and open the door.
"Yes?"
"I'm the teacher you've been asking for."

Chapter 33: *Let Man Uplift the Self*

Ding Dong. This was the actual doorbell ringing. The synchronicity of this with his writing had one word pop into his head.

... Percival...

With the normal 30-second pause he opened the door to find a man dressed in a Canada Post uniform. He handed Daniel a package and then a clipboard.

"Sign here please." There was a mixture of excitement for the unknown mail, and the twinge of disappointment that it was not his former teacher.

Walking back to his computer he tore open the envelope, pulling out a dark blue, royal looking, two book box set. 'THE BHAGAVAD GITA: The immortal dialogue between soul and spirit. A new translation and commentary' by someone called Paramahansa Yogananda. There was one little tag sticking out from one of the two book's pages. Pulling it out and opening up to the page, Daniel smiled and felt a depth of connection and presence from the words and the sender of the books.

"Let man uplift the Self (ego) by the self; let the self not be self-degraded (cast down) Indeed the self is its own friend; and the self is its own enemy – Verse 5 Chapter VI"

THE END

Post-Script

Beauty is in the eye of the beholder.
Time perceived wasted is the degenerate soldier.
Spreading derision and contempt to the
*   malcontents.*
Looking a thousand miles down the road instead
*   of the present tense.*
What's the sense? Get stuck in.
The journey's immense. Truth, luck and sin.
And it's all one-step at a time.
Not at all concerned with the reason or the rhyme.

Because I am…
Yelling and compelling for an avatars plan.
Come on down! You're the next contestant.
At the bow of the ship, fiddling with the sextant.
This thing works HOW?!
Trying to find directions from seven sisters and
*   a plow.*

Because I am…
Overwhelmed.
Not entirely sure but I think I'm the one at the
*   helm.*
Gusts of prana and I'm trying to yama the force.
Riding the waves and plotting the course.
Going straight up the stream of consciousness.
Learning to praise a little more and curse a little less.

Trying to accept being in the right place at the
  right time.
Not at all concerned with the season or the clime.

Because I am...
Well endowed.
Captain of a vessel of which I'm proud to be on
  the prow.
Gusts of prana and I'm trying to yama the force
Riding the waves and plotting the course.
There's a storm a brewin' off the port bow.
Batten down the hatches and get ready for the now.
Because it's all right in front of your face.
Here's a piece of advice laced without distaste.
Just truth.
Go back through your experiences if you're looking
  for the proof.
That this theatre of life is a constant battlefield.
Day in day out finding if it's the ego or soul that'll
  yield.
Stealing without feeling for a couple lousy dimes.
Not at all concerned with the treason or the crime.

Because I am...
Nautical.
Caught up in a trade wind blowing painstakingly
  methodical.
Gusts of prana and I'm trying to yama the force.
Riding the waves and plotting the course.
Because have you found the spirit?

The vastness of an empty mind is when you'll truly hear it.
SILENCE!!!!!....
Hear the draining waning cries of envy, lust and violence?
They're fading away.
The ebbing of the time and tide will wash your sins away.
For the next few moments, don't utter an audible peep. Envision that the ocean is the ocean, from the froth to the briny deep.
100% ridiculous. 100% sublime.
Not at all concerned with the heathen or divine.

Because I am…
Figureheading.
Not exactly figuring where this figurehead figure is heading.
But it's at the forefront of my existence.
Rushing by my ears with never-ending persistence.
Paid in full, HMS Humanity is mine.
I'm not at all concerned with the leasing or the prime.

Because I am…
Navigating.
Seasickness has passed me by and now I'm salivating.
Gusts of prana and I'm trying to yama the force.
Lusts of "I wanna's" and I'm surrounded by the source.

*Crusts of the days manna and I'm awaiting the
third course.*
*Busts of Madonna in the haven of all the world's
ports.*
I'm coming home.
The oddities of my odyssey is what you've gotta see.
I'm coming home.
The crucible of my cruise has been crucially cruel.
I'm coming home.
*Sirens sing my arriving with their siren sirening
spellbinding.*
I'm coming home.

Not at all concerned with the reason or the rhyme.
The season or the clime.
The treason or the crime.
The heathen or divine.

Because I am…
Dropping anchor.
*The ocean is my mistress and for that I'd like to
thank her.*
For her unrelenting lesson presenting.
*It's a whale of a tale but it's one that's worth
mentioning.*
That I had the scurvy, but discovered the lime.
*I'm not at all concerned with the sneezing or the
slime.*

Because I am…
Coming back from the heart of darkness.
To say that it's not so dark and not so heartless.
To say that it's not so stark and not so artless
To say that there's no loan shark and no con-artist.
Skipper of the ark and guardian of this Goddess.
I'm coming home.

Thank you Percival, a man that knows how to ride the tides and winds of change. If and when we meet again, let these words be a small token of my gratitude to you.

About the Author

At the age of 18 Paul packed two bags and traveled the world for the next decade and a half. Finding jobs such as a forest firefighter, aircraft painter, waiter, massage therapist, surf bum, treeplanter to name a few. Studying and instructing yoga since his early twenties, he now lives and works in Montreal, Quebec. www.paulbroomfield.com

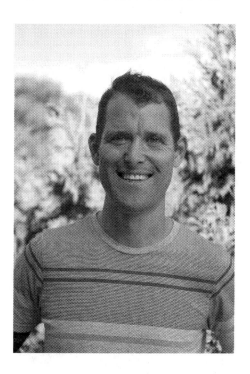